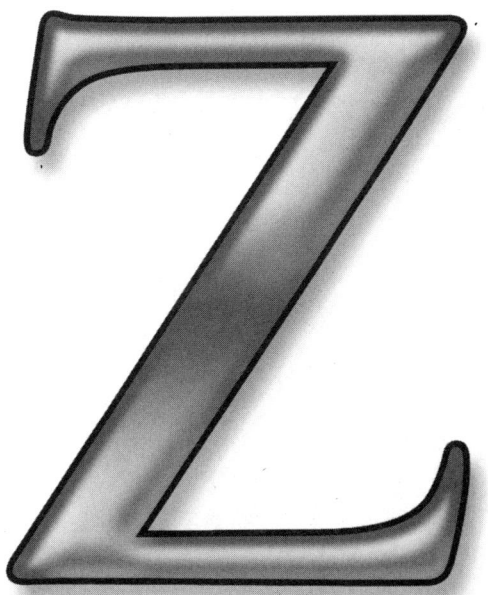

Z

the ultimate resolution starts now

healthy rapid weight loss

Dr. Bill Hopkins

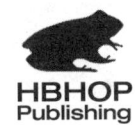

HBHOP
Publishing

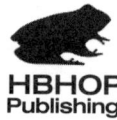
HBHOP
Publishing

The concepts and recommendations in this book are based on the author's experience. The book is the true story and practical application of how the author lost fifty two pounds in eight weeks. Although the ultimate goal is to provide a predictable, healthy rapid weight loss plan for all individuals in need, this plan in no way claims to be a substitute for your personal physician's recommendations or his/her personal advice regarding your individual health.

Z the ultimate resolution starts now

Copyright © 2006 by William S. Hopkins

All rights reserved. No part of this book may be reproduced or transmitted in any form or by any means without written permission from the publisher, except by a reviewer, who may quote brief passages in a review. For information, address

HBHOP Publishing Company
P.O. Box 51265
Bowling Green, KY 42102.

Please visit our website at www.hbhop.com

Library of Congress Control Number: 2005928631

ISBN: 0-9770045-0-3

Manufactured in the United States of America

Cover and typesetting/design by KerseyGraphics, Nashville, TN

Cartoon illustrations by Dave Owens, Gurnee, IL

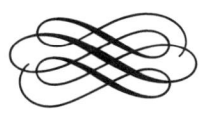

*Dedicated to my faithful wife
and our four lovely daughters*

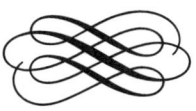

Contents

	preface	viii
	introduction	ix
A	asking yourself questions	1
B	be strict	3
C	commitment to calorie intake	7
D	diet history	9
E	examining health issues	15
F	failure is not an option	17
G	give your scale one more chance	21
H	habit forming	25
I	into the thick of things	29
J	just nutrition	35
K	killing time	39
L	lifestyle change?	43
M	mentoring	47
N	not a starvation diet	53
O	opening your mind	57
P	premenstrual water retention	63
Q	quick glance at nutritional supplements	67
R	religious assistance	71
S	serving size	75
T	teaching yourself to learn	79
U	undoing your past	83
V	variation in wardrobe	87
W	ways to win	89
X	x-treme results are possible	99
Y	you must believe	101
Z	the ultimate resolution	107
	epilogue	113
	appendix	117
	acknowledgments	118

Preface

I find it appropriate to introduce myself. I am Bill Hopkins of Bowling Green, KY, USA. It is February 1, 2005, and I am writing a book on healthy rapid weight loss.

I have recently been diagnosed with significant multi-level back problems, and I am restricted from sitting or standing more than thirty minutes at a time, bending at the waist, using my arms in an outstretched manner, and twisting my body. Although I love to tell long stories and have long conversations, my goal is to be concise. Dynamite comes in small packages.

This book is being written to share my experience with you, to encourage you, to help you, and to support you. You wouldn't be reading these words if you weren't concerned about your weight—or someone's you love. Come along. Your life is about to change. I will show you how. Introducing Z.

Introduction

Rapid weight loss was not something I had achieved in the past.

In late August, 2004, I felt a very sharp twinge in my lower back as I was walking across the living room at home. To my horror, medical testing revealed I had significant multi-level back problems. Acute and chronic symptoms were likely to be life-long afflictions.

I am physically unable to treat patients. As an endodontist, root canal specialist, my profession requires sitting for extended periods, twisting, bending at the waist, and working with my arms extended. All of these motions are physical restrictions I must respect. I will not be able to perform normally until this condition is resolved. Being physically impaired is not well-received by someone who has known physical normalcy most of his life.

Just months from being a back surgery candidate, I was desperate to heal. I brainstormed—an attempt to aid the healing process in any way I could. In early January my medical advisors were telling me nonsurgical treatment modalities were the least risky protocol four months from the onset of acute symptoms. The majority of back pain patients show improved symptoms without surgery within six to eighteen months. At that time back surgery could be the treatment of choice. With a one in four chance surgical procedures could worsen my condition, I agreed that not going there was best.

The flurry of nonsurgical approaches I came up with included healthy rapid weight loss. I rationalized my goal on

z the ultimate resolution starts now

Sunday, January 16, 2005. I weighed in that night at 232 pounds—only one pound lower than my lifetime maximum. I desperately needed to get to my target weight of 180 pounds. Weight loss could be the most significant factor in my potential recovery. I considered the importance of time in healing and set my sights on the six month mark. I had already been totally disabled from my clinical practice for four months. How on Earth was I going to lose 52 pounds in only two months?

asking yourself questions

When committing to losing weight, you must ask yourself serious questions. You cannot succeed if you do not have a firm grip on why you are overweight. What do you have to change to empower yourself to succeed?

The thought that I must lose weight quickly dominated my thinking on that special weekend in January, 2005. I realized this lofty goal may be unobtainable, but I was compelled to succeed. I was determined to give it my damnedest effort and I did.

I asked myself important questions. What could I possibly do to lose nearly one fourth of my total body weight in eight weeks with little or no exercise? How could I lose 52 pounds that quickly without starving myself or risking my health? What is it about eating that we truly enjoy? How can

z the ultimate resolution starts now

I change my eating habits drastically, still enjoy eating and consume significantly less calories? I have always believed that anything is possible if you put your mind to it. The brainstorm was blowing in.

I am not a nutritional expert; however, I know the importance of having the recommended daily allowance of vitamins, minerals, and antioxidants (currently the nomenclature is DV, daily value). To avoid eating foods I didn't enjoy, I chose supplements. I needed optimum nutrition regardless of daily calorie intake. If supplements provide daily nutritional needs, then food choices are irrelevant. Eating only foods you like is paramount to your satisfaction.

In the absence of exercise, caloric intake must be reduced to below normal or fat stores will not be burned. Intake of two thousand calories a day is recommended to maintain weight. Starting Monday, January 17th, I would consume 1500 calories per day, maximum. I would be very strict and see the results of this adjustment in one week.

My wife Jeanie and I have a digital bathroom scale. What that ordinary scale taught me in the next few weeks would change my life forever.

Ask yourself questions. Set the stage for success. Why do you want or need to lose weight?

be strict

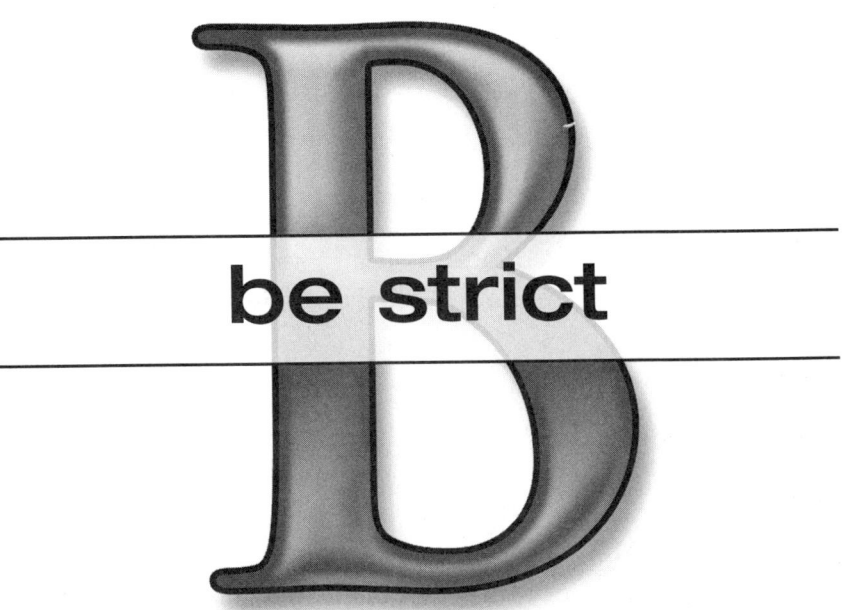

Persistence pays. Be very strict. Adhere to the principles that are outlined in these pages and you will succeed. Out of desperation, I was strict in following my plan. My career was in jeopardy. You, too, will be strict because you are so frustrated by many failed attempts at losing weight. You will succeed. I will do everything I can to see you do. I insisted on my success, and I am committed to yours.

The only thing you will lose in this relatively short term journey is pounds, inches, and bad eating habits. Pounds of body fat you have been storing for no apparent reason will be utilized as your energy source. When you reach your ideal weight, you will need to double or triple your daily calorie intake to prevent continued weight loss.

Get excited about needing a new wardrobe. You will have

Z the ultimate resolution starts now

no use for your current clothing in a few months, or less, depending on the gap between your current weight and your ideal weight—unless, of course, you would prefer extremely baggy clothes. Your eating habits will be sensible for the rest of your life.

All overeaters have a problem with self control. In a very short time, the information learned will give you the power and confidence to succeed. You will reap the benefits of this healthy plan. Your overall physical and mental health will improve. Your self-image will skyrocket.

This is not a restrictive diet. You are required to eat only foods you like. You may even expand your current food choices, taking the boredom out of eating the same old standbys merely out of routine. It is simply a matter of changing the way you eat and the way you think about eating—philosophical and psychological. Maintain self-control. It is not me that makes this journey successful. It is you. I will help you adhere to the concepts, completely change your mindset about eating, and help monitor your progress right down to the last unwanted pound. Bold statement, I know, but most diets work. It is empowering the dieter that will make this plan succeed like no other. Historically, fad diets have not overcome the mental aspects of losing weight. Welcome to Z. It is the ultimate resolution. You finally have an opportunity to be successful on the very first try.

You will not read this book and be on your own. You have proven how difficult losing weight can be. You will learn how to keep dollar costs to a minimum.

Are you committed to finally go where you used to be? Or never have been? Getting to your ideal weight is as easy as you make it, whether you have 10 pounds or over 300 pounds to lose. Again, be strict. Prove to yourself and to the world that you are no longer a self-destructive slave to overeating!

z the ultimate resolution starts now

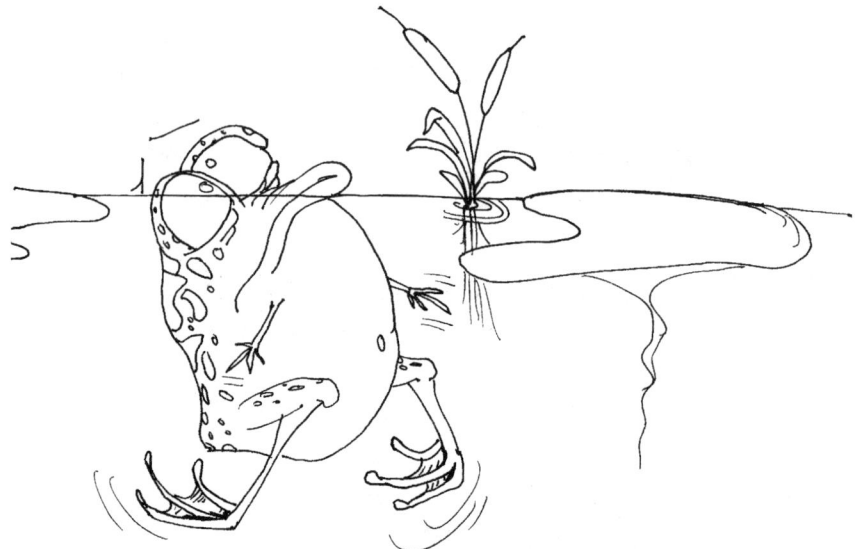

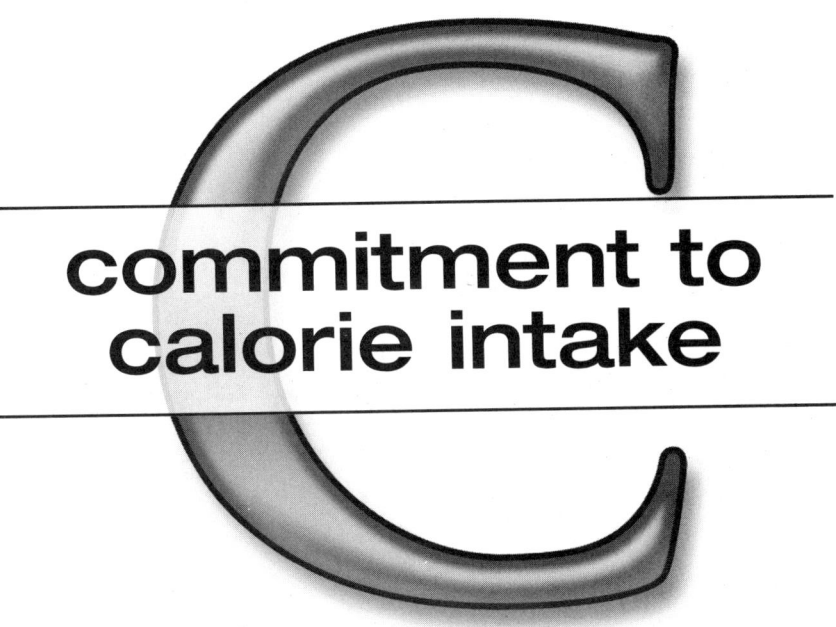

commitment to calorie intake

The food calories you consume each day are a major factor in weight loss. Commit to this concept. A 1300 to 1500 calorie intake range for three days will allow your stomach to revert to a consistent size. Overeating has caused your stomach to overstretch (distend) and to grumble when it is not full to that extreme.

The day you commit to this plan will be your starting point.

Commitment put man on the moon, cured polio, and raised the pyramids. Are you a worthy candidate to commit to losing weight? Of course, you are. Anyone can eat less. Learn and follow the recommendations presented in this book and in minimal time you will make it to Z.

Reading these early chapters does not provide you with

the information you need to be successful. Read this book from cover to cover prior to committing yourself. Along the way, I will refer you to web sites. I will not waste your time with volumes of scientific information, dietary analysis, food restrictions, or a lengthy bibliography. All pertinent information is available through your own research, internet or otherwise; feel free to explore. Once you read this entire book and all it has to offer, your mindset will be focused on a goal. You will be excited about the truths in these pages and you will commit to reaching your ideal weight as soon as possible.

You are not alone. Uncountable Americans and people throughout the world struggle or have struggled with weight control—some for their entire lives. Whatever your weight, whatever your age, whatever your country of residence, whatever language you are reading this, whatever your accustomed culture, you can set a healthy goal and reach it quickly. Reaching your ideal weight is your goal. Reaching it quickly is an inexpensive bonus.

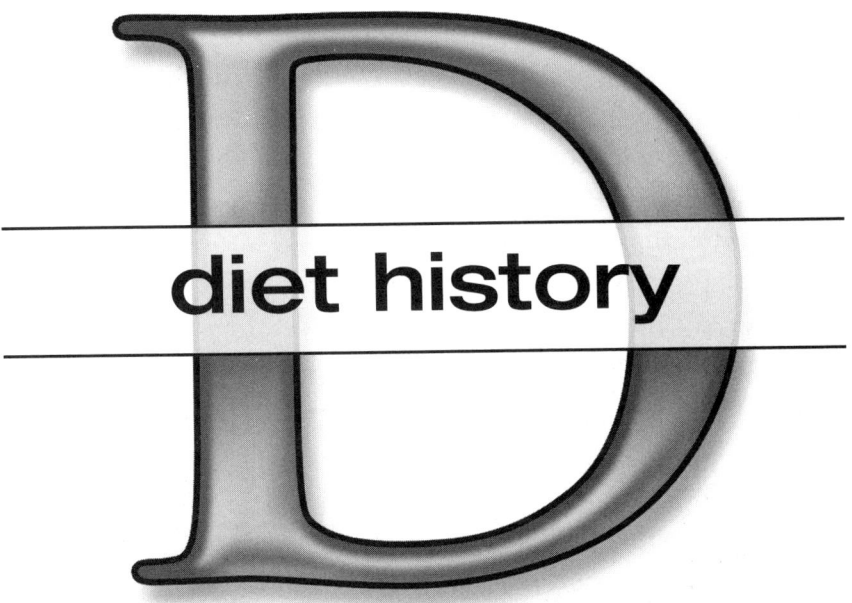

diet history

I have attempted to lose weight twice in my life. I will take you back to both times and places.

The summer before my sophomore year in high school started like many before it. I was glad to embark on another vacation from school. I loved school, got good grades, participated in sports, and had plenty of friends. I looked forward to working in summertime.

Most mornings, in the summer of 1977, I ate breakfast with the men of several siding crews. Our breakfast meeting place was a nice little family restaurant—the Blue Top in Highland, Indiana. Dad was an aluminum siding contractor. My brother and I were taught the skills of the trade as young boys. I began working with my father and his crews when I

z the ultimate resolution starts now

was nine years old. We met at the Blue Top each day for breakfast and a dose of male bonding before starting our work day.

I turned fifteen in early July of '77 and was a tad pudgy. The ring of grabbable flab about my waistline defined the fact I was overweight. The slow progression of increasing weight is a silent intruder in our lives. We put on a little at a time and eventually it shows. Gaining weight is a slow process; somehow a little change over a long period of time gets little attention from the person gaining weight. Before we know it, we are heavier than we should be—heavier than we want to be.

At one of our breakfast sessions, my dad's best friend George was sitting beside me in the booth. My routine breakfast was two over easy, bacon, peanut butter toast, and a large chocolate milk (we were regulars at the Blue Top so the waitresses stocked peanut butter in the kitchen just for us). As I was scarfing down the meal, George reached over and grabbed a handful of my excess waistline.

"Gettin' a little chubby, there aren't you, Billy? You better watch it. You'll end up like your Uncle Dan," he said.

I was silent—a little embarrassed. His comment hurt my feelings. My Uncle Dan was a Hoss Cartwright type, with a Texas beer belly that could've won a contest. George's comments really made me think.

People who love you say things that really sting sometimes. Recognize their love for you and realize they do not understand how their words could damage you emotionally. In an obscure way, the following comment made to one of my sisters when she was about sixteen was a way of saying, "I love you". Our dad said to her, "I will buy you a new MG, if you can fit in it." That was one helluva way to express his love. In case you don't know what an MG is, it is a very classy small car. Terry is 43 years old now and she still has vivid memories of that day. The comment haunts her.

At lunch the same day George grabbed my roll, I reduced my caloric intake out of embarrassment. I usually had the same thing for breakfast and lunch every day of the working summers. Lunch consisted of a cheeseburger with everything on it (extra pickles, of course), a large order of fries, and a large Coke. I eliminated some of the caloric items from the meal instinctively. No cheese, no fries and 0 calorie diet Coke. Lunch became just a hamburger with everything on it but mayo and a large diet Coke. Extra pickles, of course.

The next morning I ordered breakfast; another difficult change. Breakfast became one over easy, plain toast (still two slices), and a large milk (no chocolate flavoring). This pattern continued for the next 7 weeks and I stuck to it. What was difficult the first few days seemed easy for the remainder of the summer. Our job was quite physical so exercise remained unchanged.

By the beginning of football practice in late August I was trim and in my prime when school started. I didn't think about the results of my transformation, other than the fact that girls seemed to be more interested in me that fall. I had not gotten on a scale, except during wrestling in the winter sports season, so I don't know how much weight I actually lost that summer. Just guessing, around 20 pounds or so.

I weighed 178 pounds when I graduated from high school in the spring of 1980.

z the ultimate resolution starts now

In late 2000, Jeanie bought a copy of *Dr. Atkins' New Diet Revolution*. She has always been conscious of her weight; always tries to look her best. Our second daughter was born in the fall of 1997. Jeanie got back to her normal weight quickly after giving birth to all of our children. I have always been appreciative of her efforts. If she happens to put on five or ten pounds under normal circumstances, however, you would think by the way she responds that she had put on a hundred. I have seen numerous diet plans since I met her. I'm not so sure she ever needed one.

We met in late 1990, and married in September of 1992. I weighed 190 pounds on our wedding day; not bad for a man who went through nine years of pizza-infested post-high school education. I exercised some during those years but never had a work out routine per se. Jeanie told me she never was attracted to skinny men; that a little meat on the bones was good for her man.

After eight years of marriage, two children, and ten years in a less-than-physically-active career, I found myself tipping the scales at an embarrassing 233 pounds. I thought, "Why not? I dieted when I was fifteen." I opened the Atkins book and read it cover to cover in three days. I especially tuned in to the scientific information he so eloquently delivered, and told Jeanie I wanted to test the concepts. She had started the diet plan and immediately backed off because of carbohydrate restrictions. She loves pasta. I believe she wanted to lose about six pounds at the time. You know, get back to her ideal weight.

I, on the other hand, thought getting down to two hundred would be great. Thirty three pounds in whatever time it took would make me feel much better about me. Two hundred—I hadn't seen that number for quite a while. Now I question why overweight individuals consider aspiring to be only twenty pounds overweight or more. A completely unacceptable thought process. We feel we have such a mountain to climb just to get closer to ideal. Being twenty pounds overweight is still not healthy. Carrying unnecessary pounds is not part of this plan. If you are going down, go all the way regardless of the number! You will be at your ideal weight and your health will be optimal.

I lost 12 pounds on the Atkins two week induction diet, following the rules perfectly. I didn't stray from the principles the entire time. I love bacon, eggs, real butter. After drinking skim milk for nearly twenty years, the adjustment to whole milk wasn't too tough. Steaks galore. Cheeseburgers with real cheese. Jeanie even paid $11.99 for a 20-ounce can of Atkins Diet Bake Mix. We still have one third of the low-carb flour in our kitchen cabinet five years later.

I did lose thirty three pounds in 14 weeks. An average of 2.36 pounds per week. A pound every three days! Amazing? Don't think so. With any common weight loss strategy that goal could easily be achieved.

I missed bread. I missed candy. I missed eating a fast food sandwich's top bun. I missed crunchy foods (pork rinds are so delicious). I missed having toast with breakfast. I missed Fruit Loops. The diarrhea and the raunchy smell of excessive gas were unfavorable to say the least. I won't bore you with the shortcomings of diets that restrict you from eating your favorite foods every day. They merely set the stage for failure once you finally reach your goal.

At the time I was pleased to have reached my goal. The

metabolic changes my body underwent kept me at a stable weight for some time, even once I started eating more carbs. I slowly regained weight and tipped the scale at 215 one year later.

I maintained 215 until late October of 2003, when an accidental severe open-wound fibular fracture with extensive ligament damage led to long-term physical restrictions. Four surgeries later in mid-July of 2004, I had put on another ten pounds from my poor eating habits and lack of exercise. Later that summer a diagnosis of severe back problems led to total disability with major physical restrictions. The scale numbers continued to climb, reaching a peak of 232 pounds by mid-January of 2005.

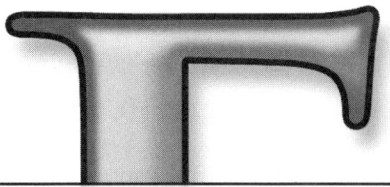

examining
health issues

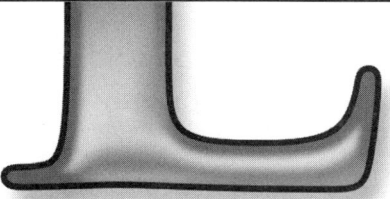

Obesity causes illness, disability, and early death. Do not enter.

It is no secret being overweight is bad for your health. A wealth of medical information is available directly correlating obesity to high blood pressure, adult-onset diabetes, arteriosclerosis, sleep apnea, high cholesterol, and joint pain. The list goes on. These facts are not myths or old wives' tales; they are reality.

Reaching your ideal weight has the potential to minimize or eliminate many of the health problems you have brought upon yourself. Don't feel guilty that you have risked good health by prioritizing poor eating habits. Reverse that process, and rejuvenate your perspective, by focusing on reaching your ideal weight as soon as possible.

Z the ultimate resolution starts now

The benefits are many, physical and psychological. Picture yourself achieving your goal quickly. What will this do for your appearance, your self-confidence, your health, and your self- image? Proving to yourself you have control of your eating habits will take you to great places. Memorable days of being trim and fit. Or will it take you to a place you have never been?

You can gain control of your eating habits. The physical and psychological changes you experience after a few weeks of strictly adhering to Z will motivate you. Enlighten you. Your mentor will encourage and guide you. I will provide more on mentors later; it is powerful stuff.

Being overweight affects us in negative ways. Get to your ideal weight. Make it your number one priority. Your life depends on it.

I ask you this question. Does the perceived pain of reaching your ideal weight outweigh the pain of your current risks: physical, psychological, and emotional? How much pain has being overweight caused in your life?

This weight loss program is a relatively short-term approach aimed at reversing years of self-abuse. I was obese on January 16th, 2005. I was fifty two pounds overweight. On March 13th, 2005, I reached my goal—in only eight weeks. I enjoyed every minute of it. What I did was more successful than anything I had ever learned. Whether or not my back problems improve as a result of weight loss is unknown at this time. In any case, I feel great about the healthier condition of my body as a whole. Consider the certainty of how getting to Z would change your life.

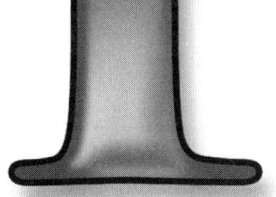

failure is not an option

There are times in all weight loss programs that we have difficulty. Changing bad eating habits can be a struggle. My goal during this process is to completely change the way you eat and the way you think about food. We all need food to nourish our bodies. How much food do we need to maintain good health? Obviously less than I used to eat. Less than you have been eating, too; you wouldn't be reading this otherwise.

Your metabolic rate will be determined early on. That information will define your daily calorie intake range. There will be minimum and maximum numbers. A range will consist of those two numbers and they will be 200 calories apart. 1300 to 1500 calories per day will be your starting range. You will ingest at least 1300 calories every

z the ultimate resolution starts now

day, but no more than 1500. You will eat three meals a day and have the opportunity to snack frequently. Your stomach will be accustomed to that level of food intake in three days. It will not be dissatisfied; regardless of what your mind is going through.

If you strictly follow the advice in these pages, you will lose weight faster than you ever dreamed possible. You will succeed and rapidly reach your goal. The definition of failure, according to Z, does not encompass whether or not this healthy rapid weight loss plan works. It does. It is proven to be healthy and rapid. You will reach your goal.

A day of failure is likely to occur at some point in time. Don't beat yourself up. It doesn't mean that you are a failure. It certainly doesn't mean you will not reach your goal. Minimizing days of failure will get you to your ideal weight faster; no question about it. It takes two good days to make up for one bad day. Food for thought: If you have seven days of success in any week, you will lose weight every day. At the end of that week you will have lost between 7 and 12 pounds. If you have six days of success each week, you will lose weight less remarkably. If you have five days of success each week, you will maintain a stable weight. If you have four days (or less) of success each week, you will gain weight. This is simple math. Three days of failure in one week takes six additional days to get back on track. There will never be nine days in one week.

Ideally, you will have no days of failure. If you can accomplish that ideal, then you are stronger than I and will be quicker to reach your goal. You must keep in mind the nature of this program. The speed is unheard of. It will teach you how to think about food. It will teach you how to eat differently. It will prove that anyone can be successful at reaching their ideal weight. You will be focused on these concepts for a relatively short period of time. When you reach your goal you will fully understand why you were overweight in the first place. Totally focus on Z. What has taken years to gain will take very little time to lose. Once you reach your goal you will never have the burden again.

I started this concept from scratch and carried it out perfectly for 12 days. At the morning weigh in of day 13, I had lost 20 pounds. Believe me, I was stunned that a number like that could be turned in so quickly. It took me 14 weeks to lose 33 pounds on the Atkins diet five years earlier. At one week (Z), I had lost 12 pounds; equaling what took two weeks with the induction phase of Atkins. On that historic Saturday, I had my first day of failure. We celebrate with food. Why do we overdo it?

My stomach had shrunk significantly. I was consistently eating much less each day than before I started this plan. I ate more than I was accustomed to, was miserably full, and I paid the price in progress. It took me two days to recover from the gain; to get back on the right track. I did nothing different from what I had previously—just stayed with the program as before. At the two week mark, I had lost 18 pounds in 14 days; could have been 21 pounds, but it wasn't. I didn't feel bad and try to eat my way out of depression. I was still very pleased with the progress.

Failure, according to Z, is weighing more on any morning than the morning before. Note that the concept applies only during the journey to your goal. Digest that definition. If your weight is less than the previous morning, you have had a day of success. If your weight is the same as the previous morning, you have had a day of success (no weight gain). If your weight is more than the previous morning, you have had a day of failure. This is not a failure of the plan as a whole.

It is your human nature not to be perfect. Try to be—I wish you good luck. When you experience a minor setback, laugh about it. Make fun of yourself for being human. Share the experience with others. Do not go it alone. Try not to let it happen again in the near future. Try not to let it happen again at all. Do not eat when you feel like you've failed. It will ruin your progress and crush your self-confidence.

When it comes to reaching your ideal weight, failure is not an option!

give your scale one more chance

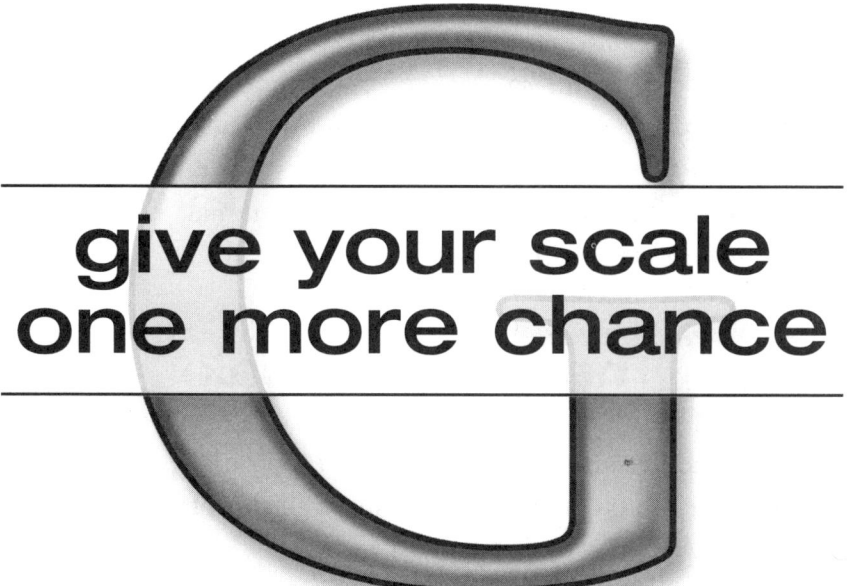

Once you have read this entire book, committed yourself to reaching your ideal weight as soon as possible, and realized the information you need is at your fingertips, you will be ready to start.

The following recommendations were derived from my personal experience and from what I have learned from people I have mentored. It is a compilation of facts and techniques that have evolved from successes and failures. Learn from it. We learn from our mistakes.

Let this information teach you the most appropriate ways to reach your goal quickly. Forget about what you have heard or read about weight loss in the past. Eliminate all social pressures of being overweight. Drive yourself to finally be successful. Others will be here for you to encourage you and to help you succeed. Every mentor in this program has been overweight, and has learned the concepts before you. Each has mastered these concepts, and has either reached a goal or is at least 50% of the way to his or her goal. An assortment of incredible weight loss testimonials have come to fruition prior to yours. Let's get down to it!

The Weight Scale

I recommend a digital scale with 0.5 pound increments. Some are available with one tenth pound increments—not necessary. An inexpensive bathroom scale will suffice if others are too expensive for your budget.

Frequent weigh ins can be a sign of obsession with weight. You may be very familiar with what I am describing.

Some are very nervous about getting on a scale. It is not their friend—too much bad news in the past. Do not be afraid. Your scale with soon be your pal, your teacher, and an empowering source of good news. It will help guide you and encourage you to be efficient.

When I developed and started Z, I weighed twice daily. This is the only time in my life I have done so. Let me explain what I learned.

In January, 2005, when a weekend of deep thought resulted in the initial concepts of this plan, I felt desperate to lose weight efficiently. On Sunday the 16th, I stepped on the scale at bedtime. It read 232—one pound below my lifetime maximum. The next morning I weighed less and I realized weight loss occurred during sleep. I weighed less when I got out of bed than when I got in bed the night before. I didn't record the number—just observed the fact. As I stayed strict with calorie intake that week, it happened every day. Each morning I weighed less than the morning before. I was strict not to consume over 1500 calories each day, but did not record the exact amount. During that week I noticed at bedtime I was 0.5 to 1.0 pound heavier than I was each morning—due to the food I ate and the liquids I drank daily. One week later, on the 23rd at bedtime, I weighed 220. I was very pleased, and recorded it. It took two weeks to lose 12 pounds in the Atkins induction phase. What I did that week was twice as fast.

Initially, keeping a log allows you to realize that each morning you weigh less than the night before. The amount you lose overnight is directly proportional to your level of hunger at bedtime. If you go to bed hungry you will maximize rapid weight loss.

Eating after suppertime prevents weight loss. I do not have a problem if people who are already at their ideal weight eat late. They do not maintain an unhealthy weight. When setting a goal and showing determination to reach that goal outweighs overeating habits, success is inevitable. Go to bed hungry tonight or tomorrow night. Weigh yourself at bedtime. In the morning you will weigh less. The instant positive feedback motivates you. During the race to your ideal weight you will long to be hungry at bedtime. You burn calories while you are sleeping. When your stomach is not full at bedtime you lose body fat overnight.

I quickly realized if I was strict with calorie intake each day I would lose weight every day. If you go to bed hungry every night, and your calorie intake is accurate and well-controlled that day, then you will drop all of your extra

z the ultimate resolution starts now

weight during your sleep. You cannot suffer from hunger while you are sleeping; you certainly cannot eat during sleep. Every morning the scale gives you good news. Every day you do your best to follow the rules. You can and you will soon know the reality of Z.

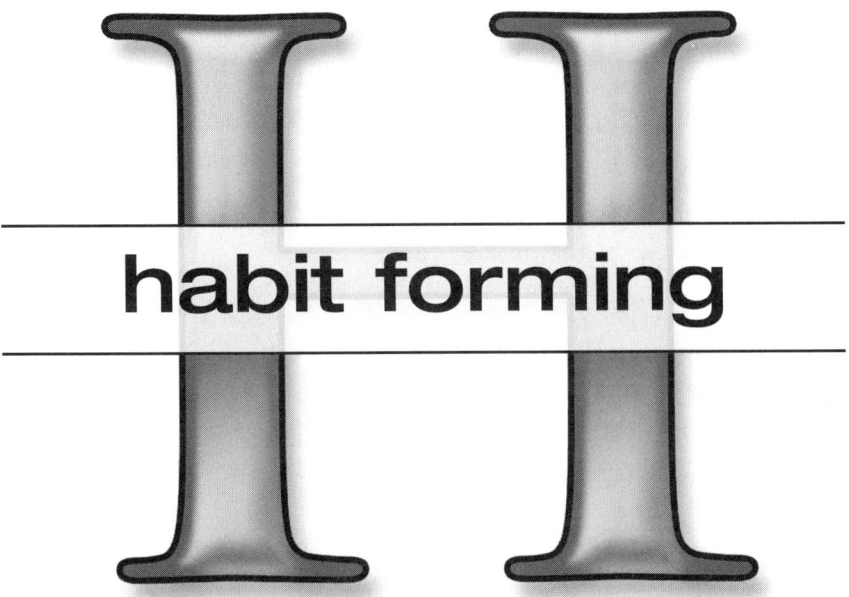

habit forming

Habits can be good or bad. You have a bad habit—uncontrolled eating. You will reverse that process 180 degrees and turn it into a good habit—controlled, sensible eating. That process alone will change your life for the better.

Some habits are good to practice daily. What are examples of good habits people have? Just for fun, I'll give you a few. Think of your own to exercise your mind, and to get a firm grip on making the things you learn from this book become items on your good habits list.

z the ultimate resolution starts now

Good habits:

- Paying your bills on time
- Kissing your spouse every time you leave home
- Helping coach your child's team
- Furthering your education

- Taking the garbage out on time
- Keeping your pets fed
- Bathing regularly
- Praying to a higher power than yourself

- Doing your best at all times
- Reading your children bedtime stories
- Laughing every day
- Brushing your teeth after meals

- Being faithful to your spouse
- Putting money in your savings account
- Keeping your nails trimmed
- Focusing on your health

Now, as a tool to help rid you of unwanted pounds, I want you to incorporate the following habits into your daily life. They are all part of what it takes to make it to Z while maintaining optimal health.

Good habits:

- Taking daily nutritional supplements
- Staying in a specific 200 calorie range
- Getting on the scale regularly to monitor progress
- Counting daily calorie intake very accurately
- Ingesting no more than 100 calories after supper

- Going to bed hungry every night
- Not feeling alone in your quest to lose weight
- Eating all day long
- Realizing exercise alone will not combat overeating
- Having three meals each day

- Eating only foods you like
- Going out to dinner and bringing a doggy bag home
- Discussing successes and failures with others
- Being completely honest about true facts
- Realizing that healthy rapid weight loss is possible

- Persisting regardless of external pressures
- Understanding the healthy benefits of weight loss
- Setting a proper example for your child and others
- Caring about the health of someone you love
- Creating your mental image of ideal weight

- Having control of your calorie intake at a buffet meal
- Leaving unwanted pounds behind permanently
- Understanding your excess body fat can be your primary energy source

z the ultimate resolution starts now

- Realizing for a short time your stomach grumbling is a good thing
- Knowing that starvation is not possible if proper nutrition is mandatory

I will do my best in the remaining chapters to convince you that all of the above are concepts to embrace. Good habits will help you achieve a healthy weight. I will encourage you to respect these concepts for the rest of your life. Once you reach your goal, you will have long-term control of your weight.

into the thick of things

This chapter answers the questions in A—the very questions I pondered that led to Z. The weekend of January 16, 2005, questions came up. That same weekend, I answered those questions as best I could. I am fortunate to have post-doctoral training in anatomy, biochemistry, physiology, immunology, and pharmacology. The philosophical and psychological aspects of this plan came from experience. I have been blessed with motivation, foresight, and persistence. The combination of these God-given traits has given me the feeling I can accomplish almost anything, if I set my mind to it.

Once a goal was in mind, the wheels began to turn. In one weekend I roughed out the concepts. Over the next four weeks, based on the analysis of my progress, I defined the rules. During that time I started teaching others about what I was doing. Through their feedback and my own experience, I refined this plan to its current strength. There is no doubt in my mind that Z will be the most popular weight loss plan in history. It is extremely rapid and extremely healthy. It strengthens the outlook of the dieter—mentally puts you in control of your eating habits. It gives you the tools you need to succeed and reinforces the concept of mind over matter. I cannot believe this plan simply came from circumstance—to you and to many, many others.

What could I possibly do to lose nearly one fourth of my total body weight in eight weeks, with little or no exercise?

It didn't take much thought to answer this question. It was obvious to me significant physical limitations would make vigorous exercise impossible. Decreasing calorie intake would be mandatory.

How could I lose 52 pounds that quickly without starving myself...risking my health?

Minimizing calorie intake, over time would require proper nutrient intake and not in the form of food. A strict supplement program would be the solution but the program would have to be cost effective. Proper nutrition would be of utmost importance if minimal food intake could not possibly supply it. The inclusion of at least twenty grams of protein a day prevents nutritional deficiency as well.

into the thick of things

What is it about eating that we truly enjoy?

Overeaters thrive on eating frequently or binging on favorites like chocolate. Unfortunately volume of food intake seems to come hand in hand with this habit, leading to above-normal calorie intake. Decreasing calorie intake often requires changing the way we eat. Important is focusing primarily on the **taste** of food and drink. Eating only foods we enjoy is of paramount importance to being satisfied. No restrictions to any food or drink. These concepts make this plan a welcome undertaking when compared to any other.

How can I change my eating habits drastically, still enjoy eating, and consume significantly less calories?

You will find portions of the answer to this important question throughout the rest of these pages. I will spend some time giving you many of the clues that help solve this riddle.

Since 2000 calories is a normal daily intake to maintain weight (depending on metabolic rate), I decided to decrease intake to a maximum of 1500 calories per day. I considered a general range of 1300 to 1500 calories per day for starters.

Staying in a specific range day after day allows the stomach to get used to a specific rhythm. In just a few days the distended stomach of an overeater recalibrates to a new size—that of an under eater. Fifteen hundred calories a day is 75% of two thousand. This is a significant drop, but not extreme. Anyone with a will to lose weight can do it. After three days maintaining this strictness, if you eat a meal like

the ultimate resolution starts now

you used to you, it will feel like a Thanksgiving feast. Don't do it; it hurts to be that full. Over the course of time—a short period of time—you will gradually shrink your stomach. Each little step convinces your stomach that less is enough. Before you know it, you are satisfied eating fewer calories a day than you could have ever imagined.

The physical act of eating includes putting food in your mouth, chewing it, tasting it, and swallowing it. You're thinking...DUH. If I am going to teach you a significant change in the way you eat, I have to start from scratch. Please pay attention.

Our tongues are incredible sensory organs. How bad does an aspirin tablet on your tongue taste? It is small. Cut it into 100 pieces, and each mini-piece tastes just as bad as the whole tablet. Reverse the situation. Chocolate frosting is delicious. A serving the size of your little fingernail tastes just as good as a heaping tablespoonful. Ninety percent of what overeaters ingest is swallowed without giving our tongues an opportunity to enjoy the taste. A wad of food being choked down is rapid calorie intake with minimal enjoyment of the food's flavor. We tend to take huge bites, a mouthful at a time, and practically swallow it whole. We taste what is lucky enough to touch our tongue on the way by. Smelling food is another way to enjoy it. Ever walk by a bakery? You can add to your pleasure at meals by smelling the foods you eat. It is a calorie-free bonus that enhances your dining experience. Maximize that experience and minimize calorie intake. When you are losing weight rapidly, it is more enjoyable to see how little you can eat while maximally savoring a micro-sized meal. You will soon agree wholeheartedly.

Take a very small bite of something you like. If a food is chewable, use your back teeth, if you have them; chew each tidbit thoroughly. All bites of food should be chewed until in solution with your saliva, if possible. Tastes great, huh? The action of chewing satisfies your brain that you are eating. The longer it takes per bite, the better. You feel like you are eating a lot when you are actually eating very little. I will give you some specific examples later.

Washing down small bites of food does not require much liquid. It is likely that the food will be mostly dissolved when you swallow it. I recommend non-caloric drinks until you reach your ideal weight. If your drinks have no calories, you can have all of your daily calories in the form of food. Make sense? If you just have to have orange juice with your breakfast, fine. Sip two ounces (approximately 30 calories) of O.J. with your micro meal. It is the taste you're after, not the volume. The same is true of anything you eat from now until you reach Z.

You must feel like you are overeating when you are not. While you are losing weight in record time, you will put food in your mouth just as many times as before, you will chew food just as much as before, you will taste food as well as before, and you will swallow at least as many times as before. You will eat only foods you enjoy. Only you know what your favorites are. Feel free to eat anything you want. Exclusions are not necessary.

z the ultimate resolution starts now

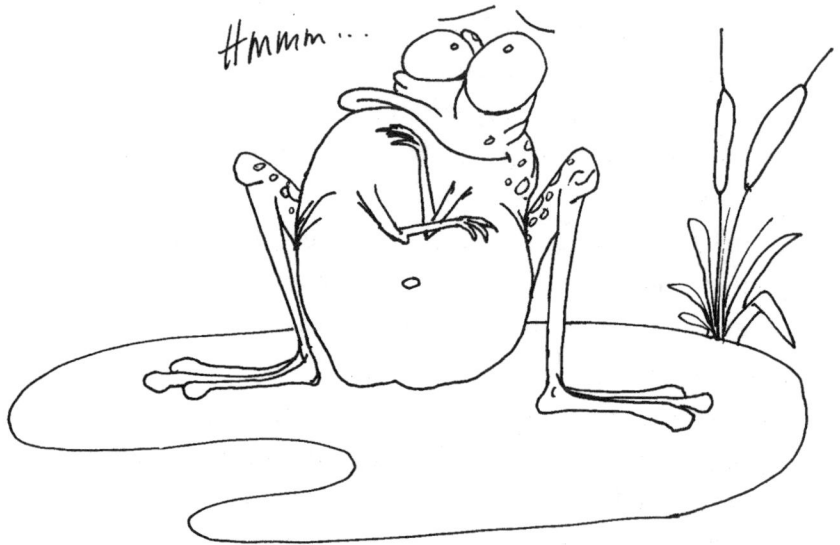

just nutrition

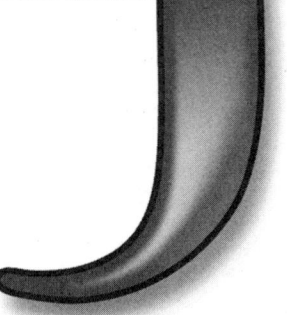

Think about this. If eating fewer calories than normal, how do we maintain good nutrition for our bodies?

It is just nutrition. Simple as that. Having the proper amount of vitamins, minerals, and antioxidants each day is essential to maintain normal bodily function. It is irrelevant whether these come from food or in the form of supplements. I have experienced the side effects—none. Let me tell you what is involved.

Realizing I had to eat much less than normal for a period of two months stimulated me to focus on what would maintain good health during that time. I am not talking about "for life" here; I am saying "only during the time" I would be consuming less food than normal. In the early stages of the process, I had no idea how few calories a day I could eat and still be satisfied. I realized that using supplements instead of food could provide the lion's share of necessary nutrients. My excessive body fat could be the primary food source. Proper protein intake is important as well.

Bears gain weight intentionally to prepare for hibernation. When they come out of the den in the spring, they are thin. You will go into a modified form of "hibernation." It may or may not be wintertime. The difference is that you will still be eating every day—-just less food. You will be eating all day long, consuming small amounts at a time. You will be eating only foods that you like, frequently. You will be losing body fat quickly. You will sleep as you normally do and lose weight while you are sleeping, just like the bear. However, you will come out of the den each day and resume your normal daily activities (all but overeating). A relatively short period of time later you will be thin, well-nourished, and much healthier.

I strongly recommend frugality in the quest for supplementation. You do not need to purchase expensive brand names or subscribe to high-priced monthly vitamin programs. Although both choices may have good intentions, they are produced by profit-driven companies. Their main objective is to produce revenues from sales.

Initially, I bought a complete multivitamin at a Kroger store, the Kroger brand. I compared it to many other brand-name products and it was much more affordable for the identical formula. I was lucky enough to catch a two-for-one sale maximizing the value of the purchase. A ten month supply cost less than five and half dollars, including sales tax.

When I got home, I read the back of the bottle carefully to assess each of the ingredients. I sat at my computer for an hour or so and researched the percent daily value (%DV) of each vitamin, mineral, and antioxidant listed. We have many, many web sites at our fingertips. I found www.wholehealthmd.com to be very helpful. I went straight to the vitamin section and took the site's recommendations to heart. I trusted the source and cross-referenced the information with other sites. They were in agreement with each other. I noted several weak spots in the supplement I bought. Other brands on the grocery store shelf had the same chemical make up. The manufacturers of these products rightfully assume the person taking the supplement will receive significant amounts of nutrients from the food he or she eats each day. Based on that fact, some of the items on the back of the bottle were supplied at levels less than 100% of the recommended DVs. Very logical. None of those manufacturers could foresee that one day a healthy rapid weight loss program would be developed. The name of that program is Z, and additional supplements must be added to the list to ensure optimum health for all participants. I will fill you in on the nuts and bolts of a supplement regimen soon enough.

Let's move on to another important concept first.

z the ultimate resolution starts now

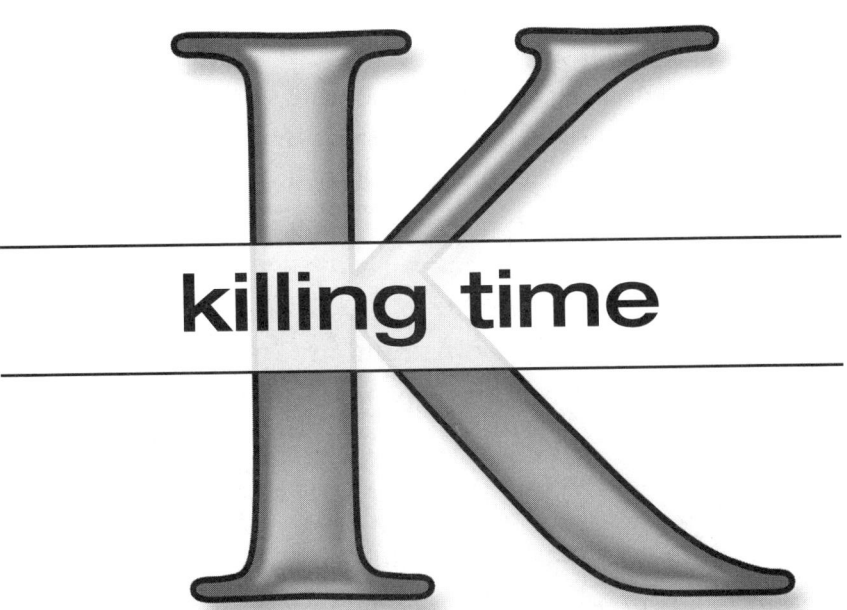

killing time

Time is of essence. I realize the phrase "killing time" usually relates to a lull or a waiting period. The concept here is this: you do not want to delay your progress for any reason. Once you commit to reaching your ideal weight quickly, get there quickly. There is no reason to delay the journey to better health. Rapid weight loss is extremely healthy, only if ideal nutrition is considered essential. I challenge anyone to disagree.

On the road to ideal weight, I decided to spread the word...share this plan on a broad scale. It is important to me that the masses have access to the information I have to offer.

I asked myself, "How can I share this information with unhealthy people globally, and have the opportunity to touch

Z the ultimate resolution starts now

as many lives as possible?" The answer is keeping costs to a minimum. People of any socioeconomic status need to be able to afford access to this plan—rich or poor, twenty pounds overweight or two hundred, from the United States, China, Canada, or Greece. I will try to reach any person who wants and needs to reach their ideal weight. It is simply my vision of what is possible.

I have seen droves of cost-prohibitive plans since making the decision to reach out to all people who want and need to lose weight. We have all seen these plans. On television. In magazines. On billboards. On the internet. It has been a learning experience for me, and has been somewhat amusing at times. Advertising has made millions for companies selling products and services of all types, including in the weight loss arena. Let me give you some examples of some very good causes that prey on the overweight individual for major profits. I will not point fingers at specific companies or weight loss plans during this examination. It is not my intent to hurt others with these comments—just to open your eyes to what consumerism can do to a society. This is not political. It is just about wasting money...your money.

A plethora of high dollar products or services are currently available.

- Buy our pre-packaged meals.
- Buy our nutritional supplements for the low price of $??.00 a bottle.
- This fat-burning pill is simply amazing...even this doctor says so.
- You, too, can be a member of our club for only $???.00 a year. Subscribe now.

- Buy my e-book for only $16.95...the price is going up SOON.
- Get our exercise gadget for six easy payments of $???.00 on your credit card.
- Only $39.95 for our new workout video.
- Burn calories and fat with our machine; buy now.
- Respond to this amazing offer now for only $69.99 and get these incredible extra gifts valued at $100.00 absolutely free.

More on the list: hypnosis, 2-for-1 sales for already overpriced supplements, online support for only 2 or 3 bucks a week, no prescription needed, before and after pictures of people who paid a high price for what should have cost very little, threats of developing eating disorders, plans that state it is unhealthy to lose weight quickly so you can continuously send additional monies for long periods of time, AAAAAHH!

They really care about your life, your family, your health, and your longevity, don't they? Steps to reach a goal are rarely stated. Detailed plans are costly. Models and actors always look perfect (as if you will look like them soon). The reality of their entire goal is this. Take money from your account, and put it into ours. Maximize profit. Period.

There are very few weight loss plans or programs that encourage you to spend less money. As a matter of fact, only one comes to mind. Z.

This profit-driven world loses sight of what reality should teach us with minimal expense. Cut costs by killing the time it takes to get to your goal. The ultimate resolution is about to unfold.

z the ultimate resolution starts now

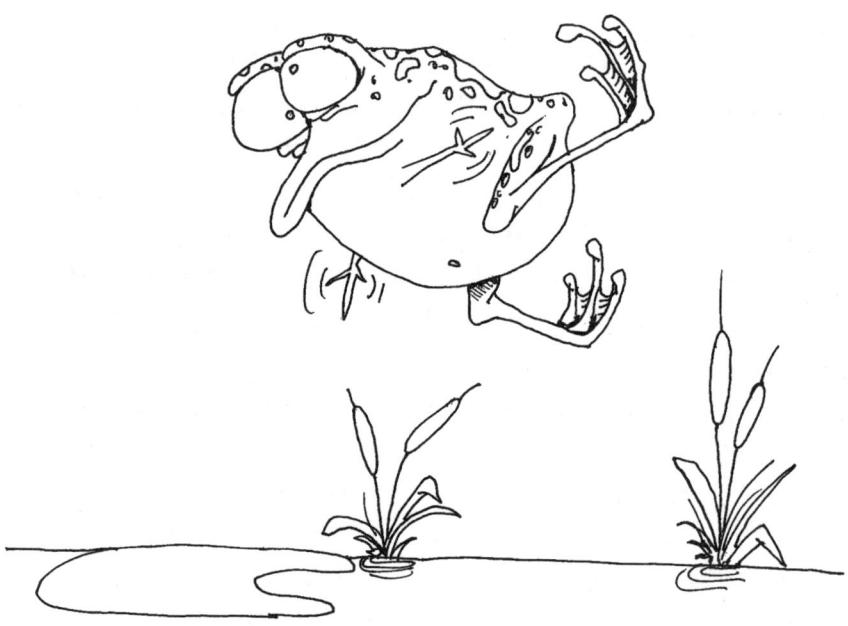

lifestyle change?

What is involved in a personal struggle to lose weight? Many programs use the term "lifestyle change."

I propose a plan to change the way you think about foods. Most diet plans are good conceptually. Do what we tell you to do, and you will lose weight. It is as simple as that.

With the variety of materials and methods that have already come across the board, why is obesity on the rise? Why is nearly 70% of the U.S. adult population eating too much? Even though the United States of America is the world leader in unhealthy eating habits, many other countries are afflicted with the same problem. Childhood obesity in this country has doubled in the last ten years. Being overweight or obese is so life-threatening that some researchers

Z the ultimate resolution starts now

are predicting a decrease in the average life span despite the incredible advances in the medical field.

We are desperate to grab this bull by the horns. We must teach each other how. Get it done. Children need to be taught by parents and teachers who have learned how—have been there, done that. Being alone in a personal struggle of any kind is difficult. There is incredible strength in numbers. Surround yourself with people who have a common goal. Help each other. I already know the power of what teaching others holds.

You need to think differently about how much you eat. Decrease volume of food consumption. On the road to Z, eat at any time during the day except the four hours before bedtime. You will learn that a stomach pang is not associated with starvation when nutrition is respected. You will soon know that when you go to bed hungry you will weigh less the next morning—every day.

People have a certain lifestyle. It has many components: family, friends, job, recreation, education, hobbies, religion, and vacation are just a few examples of what comprises a lifestyle. Changing your eating habits is not a lifestyle change. It is simply changing your eating habits. You can still keep your normal life intact. Feel free to keep the same occupation, same family, same friends, and same hobbies. There needs to be nothing different about your lifestyle. You do not have to change a thing other than your unhealthy eating habits. Everything else in your life can remain stable if you wish.

I want to make it clear that getting to your ideal weight is not about the way you look—even though our culture makes it seem that way. It is about your health, your physiol-

lifestyle change? L

ogy, your physical impairment, your longevity, and your life. I don't want you to change your lifestyle. It is absolutely my intention to change your life.

z the ultimate resolution starts now

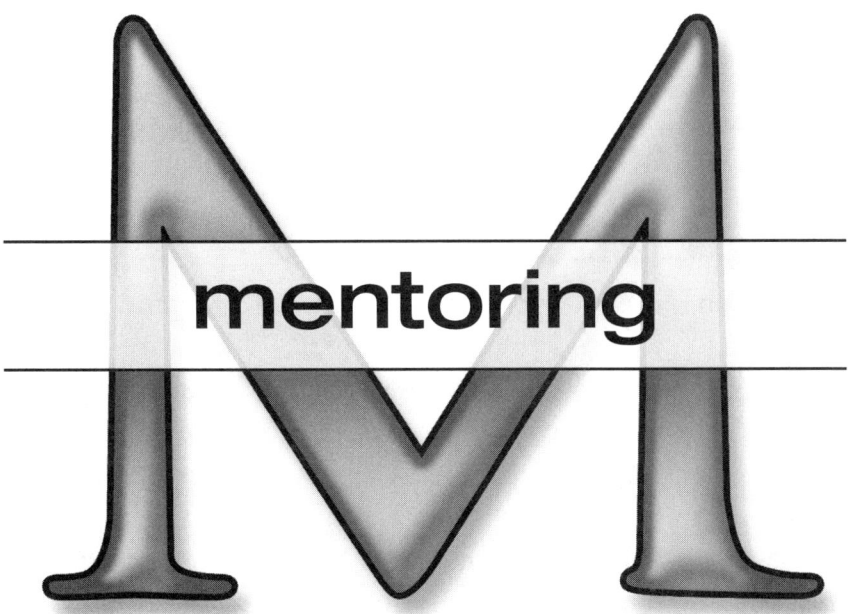

mentoring

I have always enjoyed teaching others. A mentor is a trusted teacher. Currently I am mentoring people—teaching them what I have learned. Many of them had witnessed the speed in which I lost weight and wondered how I was doing it. Word of mouth brought dozens of students to me. Some I haven't met personally. Some are my loved ones. Some are my friends.

I started an intensive series of appointments with a chiropractor in Bowling Green, Kentucky on January 17th, 2005. I was willing to do anything to improve my physical condition. At the time I was completing a series of seven epidural steroid injections which started in September, 2004. I had completed a six week regimen of physical therapy in September and October in an attempt to function normally.

z   the ultimate resolution starts now

No such luck. I was truly grabbing at straws when three different neurosurgeons recommended time and physical restraint as the best approach in early January, 2005.

A daily five week regimen of chiropractic care ensued and included treatments on a spinal decompression table. More physical therapy, electric stimulation, ultrasound, massage therapy, and physical alignment of my spine were all part of the regimen. I told my chiropractor that I was also planning to lose weight over the next 8 weeks to reduce the stress on my back. He agreed it would be a good idea. We had an interesting relationship as he watched the pounds melt away during that five week period. I shared the concepts with him during my sessions. We discussed nutrition and I stressed the importance of supplements, dietary protein, and reduced calorie intake. The combination eliminates the possibility of starvation.

I was unable to exercise vigorously. The doctor also had some weight to lose and started toying with the concepts. He and his staff watched as I lost 33 pounds during that five week time frame. He lost some weight during that time as well, but did not have the same motivation or pre-conceived time frame I had put in place for myself. He was the first person I talked with about how to lose weight rapidly. It made me feel good to share what I was learning about weight loss despite my lack of physical normalcy.

Two of my sisters had been struggling with obesity long term. When I realized what I was doing had such potential, I wanted to teach them. I wondered if women could lose weight as quickly as I was losing weight. I wanted to help my sisters—for the sake of their health. This program couldn't just work for me. I wanted to know how reproducible the results were in others.

I was able to contact my youngest sister, Debbie. I told her I had a weight loss program for her to try. When I told Debbie that I developed this program overnight, she believed in it. The girl has always looked up to me. I am eleven years her elder. I told her about my first week—twelve pounds. I included my second week—six pounds. She was excited about being my student. It was late January and Z was about to be born.

I started a chart for Debbie on my computer so I could monitor her progress. In her first week she lost 10.5 pounds. I was thrilled and so was she. Deb lost another four pounds in week two. At the end of four weeks she had already lost twenty pounds and was pleased with the rapid pace. No formal program had been laid out at the time. I was just trying to tell her how to do what I was doing—by phone and by frequent emails. Neither of us had side effects. People were soon able to see in her thinning face that she was losing weight. She was beaming and eager for more. What I was learning from our pitfalls would be powerful medicine for others I would be teaching soon.

I have a friend at church, Derek. He is a bass guitar player in our contemporary worship praise band, Cross Walk. I had developed camaraderie with him over the 15 months I had been playing harmonica in the band. He had plenty of extra weight and was about my age. He told me his physician had prescribed Glucovance, a medication to help control blood glucose levels in non-insulin dependent diabetics (adult onset). My contention is that the majority of these patients would not be taking the medication if they were at their ideal weight. Their doctors tell them they need to lose weight, but cannot prescribe to them a predictable process in which to do so. A busy physician's limited time does not allow detailed description of how to lose weight. Many of the physicians themselves are overweight or obese. Not a good situation. Medications are prescribed and the drug companies profit.

As Derek was losing weight, I had him purchase a blood glucose monitoring kit. The more weight he lost the less medication he required to control his blood glucose levels. He was able to taper off his dosage in a short period of time. His physician sees him twice a year for follow up. At his next visit, he will weigh in 60 pounds less than his last appointment and will inform his physician that he does not require medication to control the diabetic condition he used to have. A friend taught him how to do this. It cost him less than $30.00 for supplements plus the cost of his glucose monitoring kit. He is in total control of his eating habits and will be at his ideal weight in the very near future.

As a mentor, I have been blessed to be involved with numerous success stories—some still in the making. I conclude that when a goal weight is set it must be the participant's ideal weight. When one reaches a certain point, 50% to that goal, then he or she is qualified to be a mentor of this program. Control of eating habits has been mastered by that time. Perfection of recommended techniques has been mastered by that time. Confidence that was never available to these people flows from them. They want to help others because someone wanted to help them.

Mentoring benefits the mentor as well. As I was crossing the finish line in the race to Z, I was mentoring thirty to forty people. New subjects were coming out of the woodwork. I would succeed for my back's sake, but as I taught others what I knew, I realized my success would encourage theirs. I wasn't about to let them down. It motivated me to finish a winner—to prove that it could be done. They all knew this book was being written to share. Many of them will be or are mentors currently, and that is factually a key contributor to the successes of Z.

One person cannot teach the world individually—especially without a written plan to go by. You are holding the written plan. You should not be alone. It is my prediction that a multitude of Z mentors will be there to help others—because they want to. They will be touched by the willingness of others to share with them. This whole process started in south central Kentucky, USA, and will span the globe in less than a decade. I continue to have a vision of what is possible. Welcome aboard.

z the ultimate resolution starts now

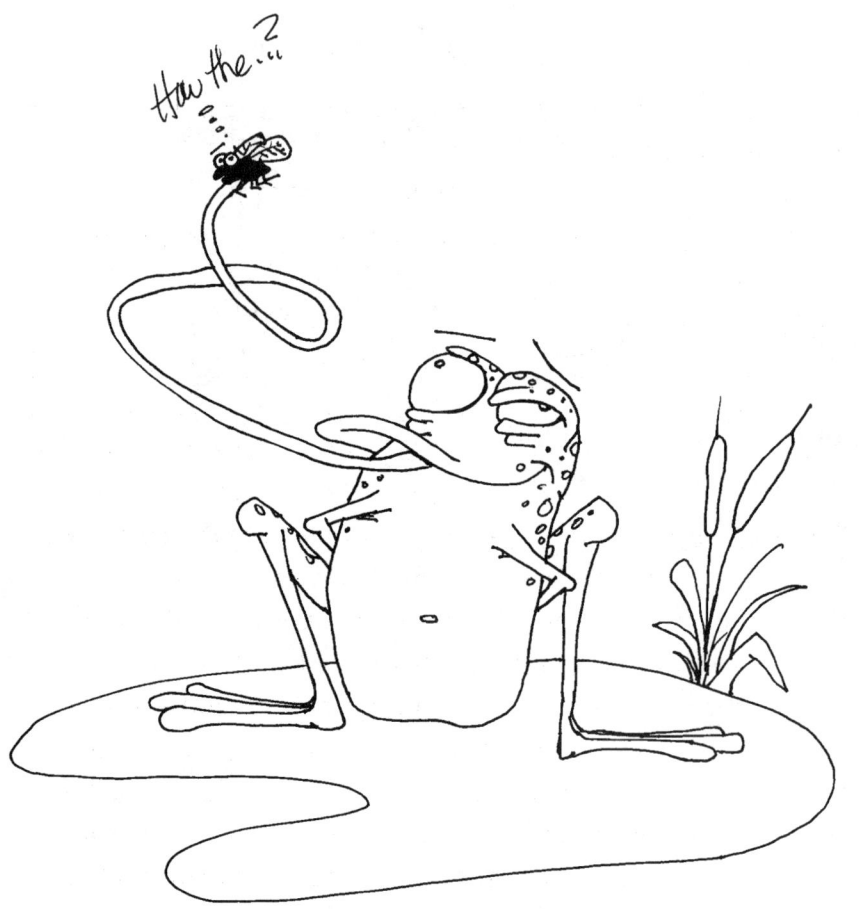

not a starvation diet

I am preparing you to lose weight quickly while maintaining optimum health. I will continue you share my philosophy with you and reset your frame of mind about eating habits. Once you realize you can be successful, you will gain control. A sense of community will lend support. You may decide to help others combat their poor eating habits.

Starvation involves weakening, wasting, or dying from lack of food. Most of us have seen pictures of starving children. They are physically weak, their little bodies waste away and they die. Not enough food to go around. When we use the phrase "I'm starving," we certainly use it out of context. Is your stomach grumbling a sign of starvation?—it absolutely is not.

z the ultimate resolution starts now

The United States of America is among the wealthiest nations in the world. We spend money for food, we eat at restaurants frequently, we consume more calories than we need to nourish our bodies, and we gain weight. Not all of us—just 70% or so. Our children are raised learning unhealthy eating habits. Our average life expectancy may decrease in time because of obesity and its co-morbidities. I ask this question to overweight individuals or individuals with an overweight child. Please answer honestly. Ponder the question. How often do you reward yourself or your child with food? Frightening, isn't it? Lives are in danger. It's time for change.

I recommend significant vitamin, mineral, and antioxidant supplementation for all participants of this program. Cost effectiveness is possible. Seek the best prices to reduce your costs. Wal-Mart and Kroger served me well. The supplements I used during my eight week journey to my goal weight cost less than $30.00. I saved more money on groceries in the first four weeks than the cost of a six month supplement regimen. Eating less food saves money over time.

Consider physiology. The body needs proper nutrition. If a person ingests 100% of what his or her body needs in supplement form every day, the need for food as a nutrition source is minimized. If that same person focuses on eating 20 grams of protein daily, the muscle wasting phase of starvation is eliminated. No weakness, no wasting, no dying. A perfectly healthy approach is in your possession.

Keep in mind that water is essential for life. All zero calorie drinks are primarily composed of water. Drink all you want; at least 64 ounces a day. When our drinks contain no calories, all daily calories consumed are in the food we eat. As we decrease calorie intake to lose weight rapidly we need to eat our calories, not drink them. This allows us to eat as much as possible even though we are eating less than we used to.

You will take your supplements daily, you will drink plenty of water, and you will eat at least twenty grams of protein every day. Your nutritional needs will be satisfied optimally. Your stomach pangs will be a reminder that fat stores are being burned efficiently. You will lose weight efficiently. You will learn that maximum weight loss occurs overnight if you go to bed hungry. The truths of these concepts will be proven, you will learn what no one has ever taught you, and you will be focused on reaching your goal in minimal time.

When you reach your goal, you will realize you must increase calorie intake to prevent continued weight loss. You will be in charge of determining your healthy ideal weight. What you learn along the way will convert your bad eating habits of the past into sensible eating habits for life. Your struggle will be over and you will never fight that battle again. What you learn on the way to Z will change you mentally and physically. Your lifestyle will remain unchanged.

Do yourself a favor. Define starvation. Think about people throughout the world who actually don't have enough food resources to nourish their bodies. They are weakened, wasting away, and dying.

z the ultimate resolution starts now

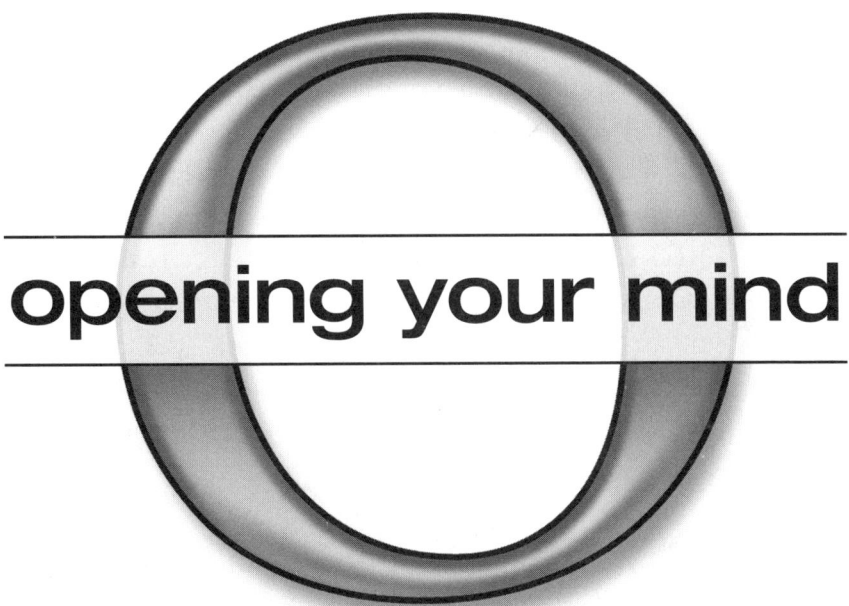

opening your mind

As you contemplate starting this program, open your mind to the changes you will employ to reach your goal. The changes will involve how much you eat, how you eat, and when you eat. What you do to reach your goal weight is not a daily practice for life. It is merely what you will be doing until you reach your goal. Once you have accomplished the journey to your goal weight, you will have the tools to maintain a healthy weight for the rest of your life.

It is time to present some essential elements of this program. I will lay out strict recommendations for success. Learn them. Live them for the relatively short period of time it takes to reach your ideal weight. Pay strict attention to the rules and follow them.

Once you have read this book, connect with a person or

a group of people to act as mentors. You may have already met a mentor, a friend or family member who has completed the program or is progressing nicely. The mentors should have control of their eating habits and should be at least 50% to their goal weight. This is a strict requirement to become a qualified Z mentor. You will not be confused and alone as you have been in the past. I have mentored many people I have never met.

Daily supplements and a minimum of 20 grams of protein intake per day are required. These two factors eliminate the possibility of starvation.

Record your bedtime weight the night before you start. For the first four weeks, you will record your weight twice a day: every morning when you rise and every evening before you go to bed. Appendix A contains a chart to log this information. It is not my intention to encourage people to get on and off the scale all day long. In doing what I recommend for four weeks, you will realize that you weigh less each morning than the morning before. You will realize that each day you gain a little weight from food and drink intake that day. The total weight gain is offset by the weight loss during sleep. Your morning weight will be less than or equal to your weight the morning before. As you know, a lack of weight gain from morning to morning is considered a day of success. These statements are true only if you stay in control of calorie intake and only if you go to bed hungry every night.

You will keep accurate record of all daily caloric intakes. Read food containers for protein and calorie content. Seek free information on the internet. Carbohydrate, cholesterol, and fat content are not relevant to reaching your goal. Do the simple math. Calculate the number of calories and the number of protein grams in your customized serving size. Suppose a breakfast pastry has 200 calories and a serving size is one pastry. Does this force you to eat the whole pastry? Suppose it contains 3 grams of protein. Do you have to eat the whole pastry because you need the protein that day? Suppose you half the pastry. This will provide 100 calories and 1.5 grams of protein. It is third grade math. You have a choice as to what you eat and how much. I recommend a variety of foods in every meal and a variety of snack choices. Eat less of each item in your meal while enjoying taste sensations from several food sources. It brings you satisfaction at each meal. Eat less of what is decadent or high calorie and more of what is lower in calories. From now on, you will be determining the appropriate amount of food in a serving size.

Drink a full glass of water or zero calorie liquid before and after every meal. You will not suffer from hunger during the day, but will strive to be hungry at bedtime every night. Again, you cannot realize hunger while you are sleeping.

Eat three meals a day, supper having the least calories of the three. Snack between meals. Your snacks should be no more than 100 calories. Have a couple snacks between meals and focus on the calorie content of each. Make sure you eat only foods you enjoy. Liquids should be zero calorie or just a couple ounces in volume if calorie-containing. You should eat allotted daily calories rather than drink them, maximizing your ability to eat foods while you are losing weight rapidly. You will be eating lesser amounts of the foods you like while maximizing the pleasure of enjoying their flavor.

z the ultimate resolution starts now

Let us look at a typical starting day, considering a maximum of 1500 calories:

Wake up.
Go to the restroom, if necessary. Record your weight.
Take bulk of daily supplements with glass of water.
Eat your breakfast within one hour.   400
After breakfast drink another glass of water.

Eat snacks between meals.   150

Drink 8 ounces of calorie free drink before lunch.
Eat lunch.   400
Drink another glass of water or substitute.

Eat snacks between meals   150

Drink 8 ounces of water.
Eat supper   350
Drink another glass of water.

After supper, your snack is minimized.   50
                                                 ____
                                                 1500

Drink zero calorie drinks before bedtime.
Go to bed hungry after evening weigh in.

Keep in mind you cannot drink too much water. Proper hydration is good for your body. If the liquids you choose to drink contain calories, then you must consider they will prevent you from eating food as you try to stay in your calorie range each day. Drinking plenty of zero calorie fluids every day fills your stomach and reduces hunger pangs.

When you are in a lower calorie range, the numbers for each of the above are downsized to accommodate your calorie range. It is important to stay in a calorie range for several days, allowing your stomach to adjust to that volume of food intake. In very little time, your stomach agrees that less is enough, and you remain satisfied despite eating less than you did in the previous range.

Every adjustment to a lower calorie range is a relatively small change. If 1500 maximum is adjusted to 1400 maximum, the change is less than 7%. A maximum of 1000 adjusted to a maximum of 900 is a 10% change.

Our stomachs can hardly tell the difference if stabilizing in a range for three to four days occurs before dropping to the next range.

You may wonder why I recommend a specific 200 calorie range every day of this program; for example, 1100 to 1300. I found it easy to stay in a calorie intake range, rather than trying to pinpoint a single number of calories every day. It gives us flexibility and choices. On any given day you may go to bed and be at the low end of your range that day. Good for you. You will benefit in the morning when your friendly scale gives you the good news. Whatever you do, don't eat 200 more calories at bedtime to get to the high end of your range for the day.

z the ultimate resolution starts now

Success will be yours if you think differently about food and why we need it. It is used to nourish our bodies. You will be using a new philosophy about eating to actually learn to under eat for a period of time, reversing the process that is responsible for your current problem—overeating. We as overeaters must still feel like we are overeating, even though we are under eating until we reach our goal. Are you ready to make some changes? If you do, you will never regret it.

premenstrual water retention

Ladies, one fact of life you will not escape is being female. A woman of child-bearing age retains water weight prior to menstruation, preparing the body for pregnancy. This is a healthy physiological process of life and is simply part of being a woman.

Having a monthly visitor frustrates women consistently and most language I have heard from women regarding premenstrual water retention, or even PMS, is negative—very negative. Realize the intricacies of nature. Respect them. You may be thinking, "That's easy for a man to say." I will leave additional choice words to you.

Rapid weight loss will be delayed by water retention phenomena from any source. Congestive heart failure patients frequently have swollen ankles. Some medications,

z the ultimate resolution starts now

particularly long-term steroid therapy, lead to water retention and weight redistribution. Hormonal imbalances can play a role as well. Premenstrual water retention is likely the most common of these, affecting a significant percentage of the population worldwide.

The weight loss data from the women I have taught demonstrates the fact that 8 to 12 days prior to menstruation, weight loss potential is greatly reduced or stopped. Water is retained. The physiology is controlled via female hormonal changes. Minimal progress is expected for women with child-bearing potential during this time. Two to three days into menstrual flow, rapid weight loss restarts. Mother Nature's need for water retention ceases. The next two to three weeks is your optimum time to make significant progress. Hence, an average of 10 to 15 days a month is involved in slowing of progress due to premenstrual water retention. Expect it to happen every month. Do not worry about it. These days cannot be considered days of failure if you stay in your calorie range. Count on it happening and stay on course. Starting your period will be a monthly reminder of your maximum potential to lose weight—the numbers begin to drop quickly again three days after your menstrual flow starts.

I remember the old saying that women have a harder time losing weight than men. From observation of the many women who have depended on me to help them lose weight, the truth of that old saying was served to me on a silver platter. Now I know premenstrual water retention is responsible for making the statement a true fact. Women do have a harder time losing weight than men; however, nothing should stop women from reaching a healthy weight as quickly as possible—especially not a natural healthy process she cannot control.

I was finally able to convince my beloved sister Terry to try what I was doing. I wanted her to overcome a lifetime of obesity. Her weight had been a struggle for her since childhood. In early email correspondence with her and many other women, I learned much about thinking of overweight women. I learned most importantly that many people feel that losing weight is a hopeless struggle.

I quote her directly:

> "I have to have the right mind set and right now I'm just not there. I know myself very well and I don't want to set myself up for more failure. I don't mean failure in the sense that your regimen won't work for me, but I have not been able to stay focused or strict with my caloric intake. I will fail in that area and I don't want or need to feel bad about myself any more. I've spent too many years trying to lose weight and failing."

My heartfelt response included this sentence:

> "Eliminate the words I will fail from your vocabulary permanently."

This fine woman is very close to me. She is my elder by one year and two weeks. I respect her. I use this example to display the commonality of the thoughts of people who have struggled and lost the battle in the past.

All women I have communicated with have similar dread

in their words about weight loss. I am not so sure men care much until they have a first heart attack—maybe not even then. Women and men are from different planets. They think and behave differently. You've probably read that as well.

The ladies I mentored in the early stages had some interesting thoughts about the lull in progress associated with premenstrual water retention. Some typical examples include the following:

> "It's the usual waiting game for me."
> "I feel like a water balloon."
> "I know how much I've hated this
> brick wall I've been leaning on."
> "I've been in the game long enough
> to know about all the set backs
> and hurdles."
> "I feel like the tortoise, not the rabbit!"

Prepubertal girls, postmenopausal women, and all males do not have the issues with premenstrual water retention as women of child-bearing capacity do. Please avoid frustration by realizing physiological facts. Look forward to losing weight rapidly again in the near future. You can still get to Z as quickly as possible. I smile as I quote an old commercial, "It's not nice to fool Mother Nature." She knows best.

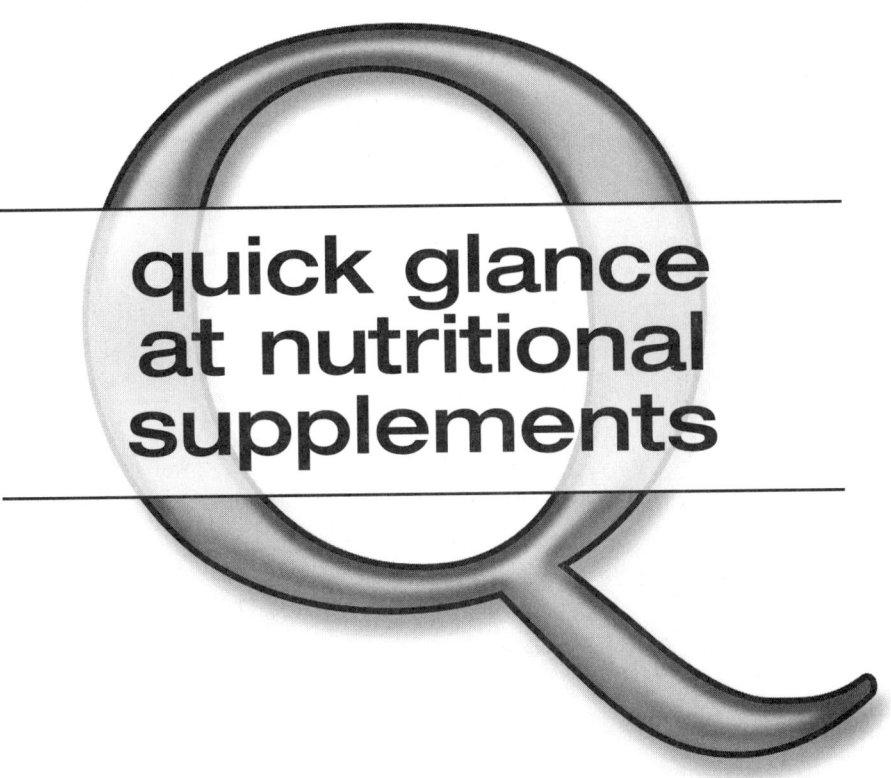

quick glance at nutritional supplements

I have described the processes of why and how I added dietary supplements to this program. You need to purchase supplements prior to starting the short journey.

I will list the supplements I personally took daily during rapid weight loss. I recommend a minimum of 100% DV of the majority of items on the back of a multivitamin bottle. See what is contained in the multivitamin you choose and add supplements as necessary. An antioxidant preparation in addition to your multivitamin will provide some of the following recommended daily supplements at appropriate levels. Add the others that are lacking. Spend as little money as possible. Generic is fine. You already know where mine

Z the ultimate resolution starts now

were purchased, Wal-Mart and Kroger.

The following are included in the list of supplements I added to a complete multivitamin daily to maintain optimal nutrition while losing weight rapidly:

- Calcium 1000 mg / Magnesium 400 mg / Zinc 15 mg (take one tablet 3X per day with meals).*
* All others were taken with a glass of water after morning weigh in.
- Complete Multivitamin
- Vitamin C 500 mg
- Vitamin E 200 IU
- Selenium 200 mcg
- Beta Carotene (equivalent to 25,000 IU VitA)
- Biotin (one quarter of 1500 mcg tablet daily)

This combination of supplements was derived from information in the vitamin section of wholehealthmd.com and cross-referenced with several other web sites. If desired, customize your regimen after relating your specific health issues to the supplement recommendations advised for a particular ailment.

Note that some antioxidant preparations may eliminate the need for additional Vitamin E and perhaps others, minimizing the total number of supplemented pills per day. Read the labels; design your supplement regimen accordingly. Be sure to include all of the above specifically. They could be the ultimate combination of supplements to allow healthy rapid weight loss. Perhaps eventually other scientists will prove the theory in the laboratories.

I recommend that you purchase an inexpensive plastic

quick glance at nutritional supplements Q

pill organizer that provides space for each day of the week. Load your supplements into the container once a week to save time going through multiple bottles every day. I found that multiple pills taken at one time wash down easily with a glass of water. Initially I took each one singly. Realizing I used to swallow such huge bites in the past, I started taking all morning supplements in one swallow as well. You will be surprised how easy this is to perform. It will save you time as well.

The benefit of supplementation while decreasing caloric intake is twofold.

First the physiological component will be discussed. Our bodies recognize each day that we have ingested at least 100% of many necessary vitamins, minerals, and antioxidants. Consequently, as 20 grams of protein are ingested each day and water intake is optimal, daily nutritional requirement is met and the body lacks the signals to go into starvation mode. It is virtually impossible. Therefore, as calorie intake is reduced over time and nutritional requirements are already accounted for daily, the biological machinery for utilizing fat stores is activated to its maximum potential. As less food is ingested, fat stores are utilized. We confuse our bodies into assuming significant food intake represented by optimum levels of water, nutrients and protein. Its sensory machinery is convinced we are eating much. Whatever we add throughout the rest of the day does not contribute to our nutritional needs significantly. The needs have already been satisfied. As less food is ingested, more fat stores are burned and weight loss progresses rapidly.

Secondly, the psychological component of nourishing our bodies is satisfied. We know in our minds that nutrition is

Z the ultimate resolution starts now

being respected fully. We know that water intake is optimal, vitamin intake is optimal, mineral intake is optimal, antioxidant intake is optimal, protein intake is optimal, and daily calorie intake is not a significant factor nutritionally. Regardless of an occasional grumbling tummy, we have fortified our bodies successfully by respecting nutritional needs each day. Although we now know that volume of food intake is negligible, we strive each day to feel as if we are overeating when by design we are not. We can now change our eating habits to satisfy our personal need to eat and enjoy foods each day without disregard to daily caloric intake. We will be eating less on purpose.

You will be responsible for accurately counting your daily caloric intake. Accuracy and truth are mandatory.

Jot the numbers down to insure accuracy. Read the containers. Get out the measuring cups. Use level tablespoons. Study the calorie content of your favorite foods. Customize your serving sizes to your liking. Measure your portions accurately. You must carry out these procedures to successfully comply with the recommendations. You will learn to respect your eating habits and to have control of what and how much you eat each day. It is all up to you.

At a glance, water intake, nutritional supplementation, and dietary protein intake are equally important factors in maintaining excellent health as rapid weight loss occurs. Keep them all at the top of your priority list and Z will be welcoming you in the near future.

religious assistance

The majority of people in this world have a religious perspective in their lives. Since ancient times people have worshiped and prayed. The power of prayer has never been discounted as a factor in solving many of our concerns in life. Our religious beliefs give us strength in times of trial and give us hope during difficult times in our lives.

If you believe in a power higher than yourself, look to your faith for assistance in accomplishment. If you do not have faith in a higher power, please consider the positive changes in your life faith could expose.

Discuss your weight problem with your pastor, priest, or other religious leader in your life. Put in a prayer request at your place of worship. Ask for others to pray for your strength in accomplishing your weight loss goals and achieving better health. Prayer teams will support you. As an individual, pray from your heart. Use the omnipotence of your Lord to help you and others commit to reaching ideal weights. A church family exudes genuine concern and support for its members. People help others just for the sake of helping them. The goodness multiplies and has potential to be far-reaching.

I personally follow Christ. My faith stems from early childhood and was initiated by the influence of my mother. Generations of our family have taught each other the principles of the Bible, the need for worship, and the power of prayer. In the life of a Christian, faith is a process of growth. As we continue the Christian walk through this life, we realize that faith is not stagnant. It is a dynamic progression. The process of developing and maturing in faith is a lifelong undertaking. As in striving to lose weight, faith requires commitment.

I realize across the globe there are many factions of religious belief. There are many gods being prayed to for strength. Your religion can assist you in reaching your goals; it could be the one part of the equation that empowers you to succeed. Do not underestimate its power. If you are a religious person and you cannot admit your vulnerability, your neediness, and your humility, then you have a problem with your depth of faith. You may just be going through the motions. If you cannot find strength through your religious beliefs, then your religious beliefs may be superficial or too shallow.

On the other side of the coin, depth of faith can be empowering in all aspects of your life. Customize your religious perspective to help you commit to losing weight. Pray

religious assistance R

about it. Generate the support of others in the church family. They will help you overcome your struggles.

If you have no religious influence in your life, use all other aspects of this book to succeed. If you fail, find religion. It is the very nature of how this book has been created. It is not my doing. It is truly a gift from God.

All people of the civilized world will have access to this plan in due time, regardless of their cultures or religious beliefs. Again, spreading the potential of this program far beyond Bowling Green, Kentucky is merely a reflection of what I believe is possible. I pray for this program to come to full fruition for the benefit of many. This prayer is being answered as I write.

z the ultimate resolution starts now

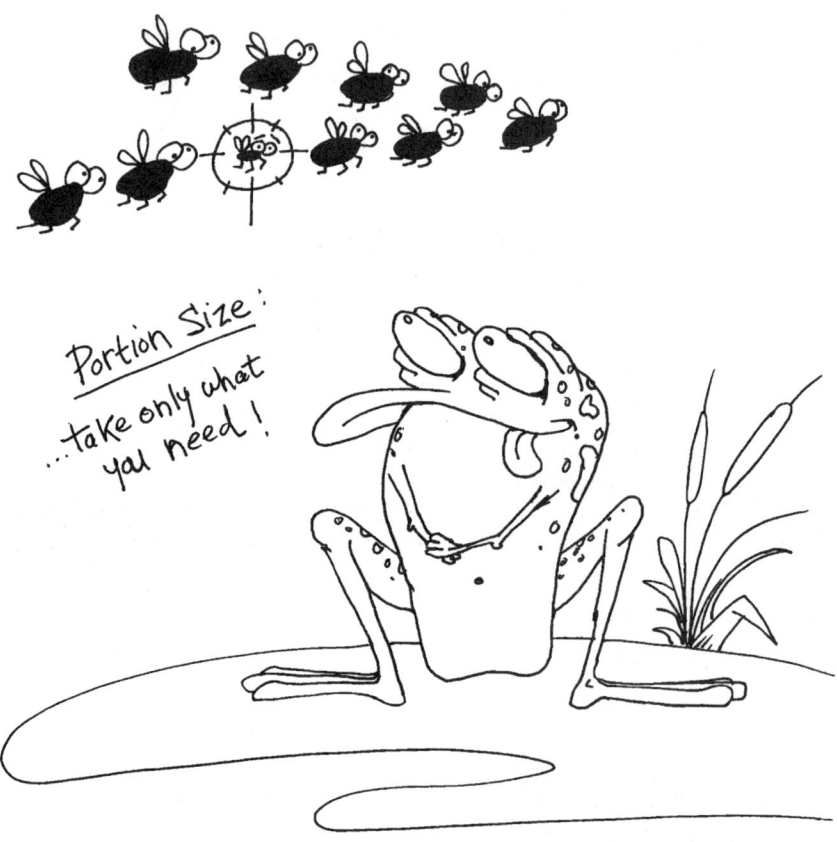

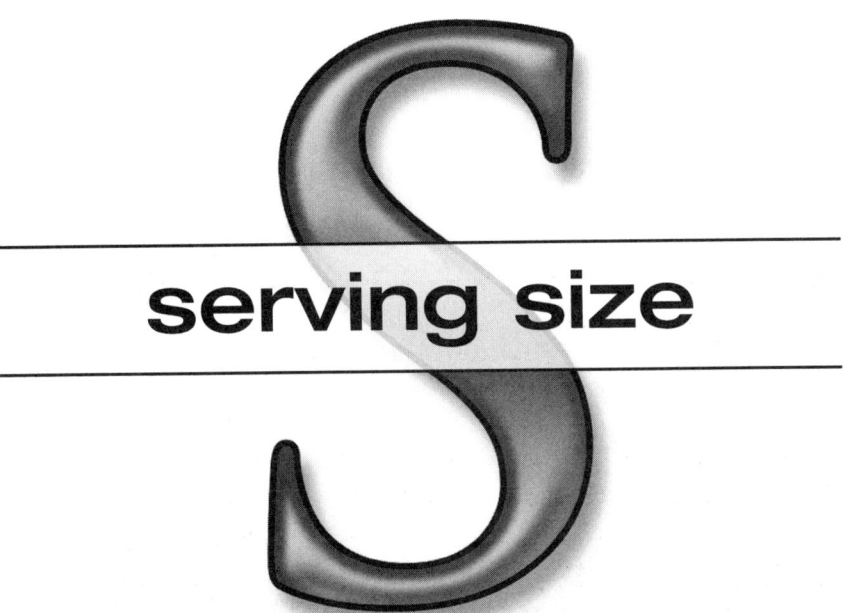

serving size

Paying attention to serving sizes will pay you dividends in weight loss. While the scale numbers are going down you are responsible for determined what, when, and how you eat. The **what** consists of your favorite foods, the amount of each you incorporate into a meal or a snack, and the variety of taste sensations you desire.

As you decrease your calorie range throughout this program, you must be in control of the serving size of the foods you eat. The numbers on a box or container can be assumed to be accurate. If you do not have a guide, then in your mind's eye the calorie content of a particular amount of food you serve yourself must be as accurate as possible. Overestimate the calorie content of foods if there is any doubt; for example, while at a restaurant or a potluck dinner.

z the ultimate resolution starts now

This will protect you from extending beyond your current calorie range that day. Predetermine how many calories of any food you are planning to eat and serve yourself exactly that amount. Only you know what and how much of each item you are eating. You must be accurate in determining or estimating all caloric values of the foods you choose.

Put the rest away if at home or walk away from the buffet. Minimize temptation to overeat. You are not going to eat any more calories than you plan to eat, so you must give yourself every psychological advantage. If the food is put away after you establish your serving size, then it is out of sight (not particularly out of mind). If you get away from the buffet before loading the extra cookies on your tray you are doing well. You could go back and reopen the box and have just a few more graham crackers. You could go back to the buffet and reload your plate. Don't do it. You have predetermined how many calories you are preparing to eat, and you are committed to eating exactly that number of calories during the meal. Drink a full glass of water or zero-calorie substitute before and after you eat. You will be satisfied and your stomach will be full although caloric intake was accurately respected. Similar minor changes in behavior will assist you in changing your eating habits. A few simple changes will make a difference in your potential to lose weight efficiently. No mentor can make you eat less. Commitment to reducing calorie intake is solely the responsibility of the dieter. Be as strict as possible.

Eating only your favorite foods brings satisfaction. Serving yourself accurate calorie amounts is enhanced by focusing on measurements. Are you serving level teaspoons or tablespoons of food items or heaping serving sizes? A measuring cup is helpful for accuracy. Did you have a bowl of cereal with milk for breakfast? Note the calorie content and amount of serving on the container. Did you eat one half cup or a cup and a half of cereal? Did you have 4 ounces of milk or 8 ounces of milk in the bowl? Making accurate determinations of your caloric intake is necessary to ensure you remain in your calorie range each day. Make a habit of recording the caloric value of all foods you eat and drink each day. Jot it down in a notepad to be sure nothing is omitted. Accuracy and honesty are keys to success.

As you lower your calorie range with time, continue to eat your favorite foods but concentrate on eating lesser amounts. Lower your total caloric intake over time as your stomach readjusts to the lower calorie intake ranges. Accustom your stomach to a specific calorie range by remaining in that specific range for at least three or four days. If you drop calorie range every two weeks, weight loss will not be as rapid.

Weight will continue to be lost as you eat less. Go to bed hungry every night. Sleep without hunger and wake up looking forward to eating breakfast. Drink zero calorie drinks. During mealtime it is much more satisfying to eat food calories than to drink them. This change gives you maximum potential to be successful. You must maximize that potential to satisfy yourself during meals and snacks. Ideally, all calories consumed should be eaten regardless of what calorie range you are in at the time. Drinking significant calories during this plan deprives you of your ability to eat. Learning to control your calorie intake while respecting nutrition is the most important component of this predictable plan.

Experiencing a variety of taste sensations also leads to

satisfaction. Serve yourself small portions of several foods while respecting calorie content. You choose what and how much of each. You can have larger portions of low-calorie foods or a small portion of something higher in calories. It's your call. From experience I know at times I preferred a one inch square of chocolate cake instead of a half jar of dill pickle spears, a Girl Scout cookie with 2 ounces of skim milk instead of a dozen pieces of shaved deli ham, or half a candy bar instead of two eggs. Without question a distinct advantage of Z is eating only what you prefer. It is your choice. Only you can determine your serving sizes and what food each contains. You have maximum responsibility and control. Pick and choose wisely, satisfy your taste buds, drink plenty of liquids, satisfy your stomach, and satisfy your scale.

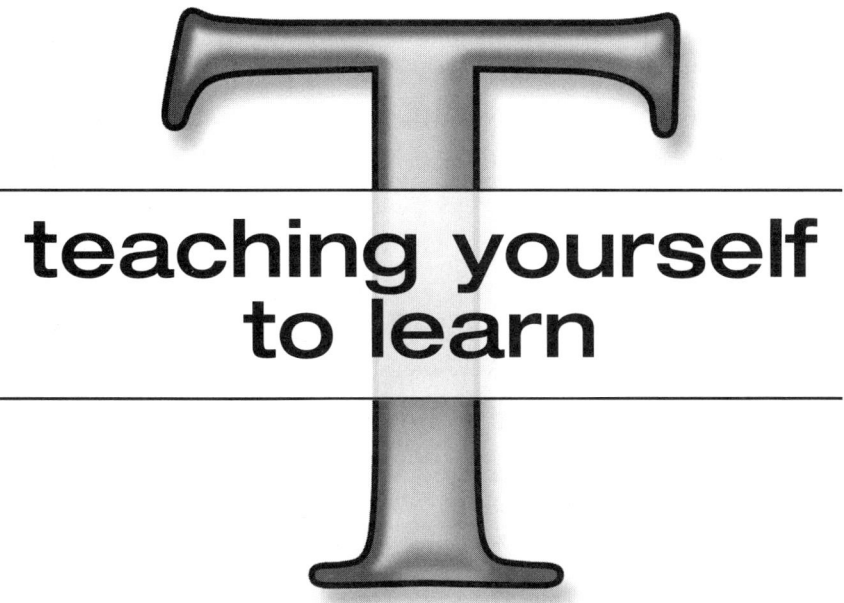

teaching yourself to learn

Throughout our lives we learn, usually from our own mistakes. Have you ever noticed when you have a problem with a certain task, it motivates you to accomplish that task? I am fortunate to have strong problem-solving ability. I have had this trait since my youth.

In week four of my journey I only lost two pounds. I had been strict around 1300 calories a day. Eating after supper became a notable problem when comparing the day to day weight loss numbers I recorded. I was eating less food during the day; saving calories for the evening. I was just over 50% to my goal at that time and was still quite pleased. I decided that minimizing calories after supper and going to bed hungry every night would yield the best results possible. That decision was correct. I hypothesized that decreasing calorie intake consistently would lead to continued positive results. I dropped my range to 1000 to 1200, knowing I had been hovering close to 1300 calories a day the week before. That adjustment was a small percentage change in overall calories allowed daily. I just ate a little less of my favorite foods per serving. Remember you alone are responsible for the serving sizes you prepare to eat. I was learning continued weight loss was possible only if I ate less. I was teaching myself and was learning from others as I mentored.

Three days later I dropped range again at 900 to 1100. My stomach didn't show much difference by its response, but the scale numbers did. I focused on eating my smallest meal in the evening. After-dinner snacks were minimized at this time. At five weeks I had lost 33 pounds, was eating around 1000 calories a day, and drinking zero calories a day. I was not hungry all the time. I drank plenty of water and diet soft drinks to keep my stomach full. I wanted to be hungry at bedtime every night. Consistency was a must. I wanted to see a lower number on the scale every morning than the morning before. My pants were practically falling off of me. Wearing a belt was a necessity. I was using holes in my belt that I had never used before.

The determination to succeed was strengthened by leading others. I was determined to prove to others they could persist as well. As data came to me I analyzed it, coached and encouraged the sender, and I continued to learn. I had three weeks to go and nineteen more pounds to lose.

Our babysitter Amanda got on board. She noticed my physical changes and wanted to know how I was doing it. I offered to teach her as long as communication was frequent and via email; just like what I was doing with my sisters.

Amanda is very bright and taught herself to be creative in her meal packaging and planning. Preplanning calorie amounts allowed her to control exactly what was in front of her at mealtime. She was persistent. She was teaching herself how to change her eating habits, and how to do these things without regard to social pressures. Specific amounts of calories were contained in each of her pre-packaged lunches. People around her were wandering what she was doing. As others noticed her slimming face and body, they asked the old weight loss cliché, "Have you been losing weight? What have you been doing?"

Carol, the mother-in-law of a friend, heard of what I was doing and showed great curiosity. I met her poolside at my buddy's home on a summer day. We spoke at length about what I was accomplishing. A registered nurse for many years, she listened intently as I discussed the concepts of this plan. I told her all of the forty or so people I was mentoring at the time had computers at home. She told me she and her husband, Pat, did not have a computer. They lived a good piece from Bowling Green and I realized we could not communicate as well as I would've liked. In light of that, I offered to get the advice pages I emailed to others who were learning about Z to her. I told her to call me any time if she had questions. I considered whether or not a few pages of information, the concepts of this book in a nutshell, could help her without frequent communication with a mentor. She received the information, which was sent to her daughter's home electronically as a matter of convenience, and she put the advice into action. Carol wanted to lose about 50 pounds at the time to get down to an ideal weight for her age and body type. As a nurse she knows what a healthy weight is, but had struggled as so many do in accomplishing the task. A few weeks later I saw her again at the poolside. I had no phone calls from her during that time for additional advice. She told me she was very pleased and was moving nicely in right direction, breaking barriers she could not accomplish through her many years of attempts with diet plans and available weight loss products. With over 90,000 weight loss or exercise products on the market currently, I wonder why obesity is on the rise world-wide in adults and children. It is intriguing so many people are trying so hard and not getting it done, regardless of cost. I had the opportunity to be alone with Pat in the house that day. He was very pleased as well. He wasted no time in commending what Carol was doing to lose weight. Pat saw her progress firsthand. I quote the good man, "She's doing great, Bill. I haven't seen her this excited in years. This plan of yours really works!" It touches me to see the progress people are making. I talked to her recently and she was already 40% to her goal. She is teaching herself to learn a new way to get it done. Z is changing her life.

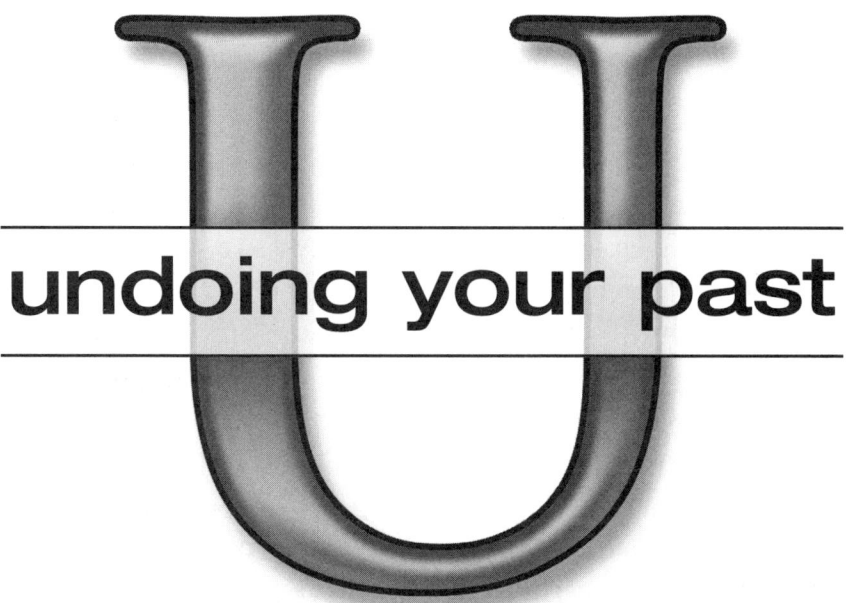

undoing your past

Old habits are hard to break. You must be able to institute changes in your eating behavior to be successful at weight loss. Overeating is a daily routine in the overweight and obese population. Most of us do it regularly and weight gain is the result. Changing the way we used to eat proves that we have learned. I reiterate a comforting fact. Once a person reaches his or her ideal weight, calorie intake must be increased to prevent continued weight loss. What you do to reach that goal does not continue for the rest of your life, but the lessons you learn will not be forgotten. This plan is designed to allow one to learn how to control eating habits strictly until a predetermined goal is reached. That goal is one's ideal weight. Reach your goal as quickly as you can. Once you realize how little time it takes with true commitment, you have a powerful boost mentally. You realize that persistence pays and that consistency yields phenomenal results.

I remember how I ate before I set the eight week time frame to reach my goal. I overate routinely, and spent little time ingesting large amounts of food. I wasn't stuffed at all times. My stomach was used to a consistently high volume of food intake; much more than I needed to nourish my body. I ate more food than I needed, and over the years I gained weight slowly. I was obese when I designed this plan.

I was lucky not to have health problems of major significance due to obesity. In retrospect, I wonder what affects the extra weight I was carrying may have had on my back problems. I mentioned earlier, do not beat yourself up for risking your health. Whatever problems your weight has caused in your life can be minimized or eliminated when you reach your goal. If you have no medical problems as a result of being overweight or obese, it is likely that you will develop a problem at some point in time. Change your eating habits now as a preventative measure.

My back may never be same due to the complexity of its problems; however, I am certain my weight will not be a negative factor regarding this man's health.

After experiencing constant back pain for four months and following non-surgical recommendations for relief that did not come, I was concerned about my blood pressure. Early in the onset of disabling symptoms, my blood pressure rose. I had not experienced high blood pressure throughout my life until that time. With continuous back pain and sleep deprivation becoming a part of my life, my physicians were attributing the rise in blood pressure to those recent medical issues. Four months after my back failed, at the chiropractor's initial examination, my blood pressure was dangerously high. Three weeks later, after losing 24.5 pounds, I asked the nurse to check my blood pressure. I was curious. Pain levels had not decreased, nor had I been sleeping more than four hours at a time. Nothing had changed except my weight. I was physically unable to exercise vigorously. At that time my blood pressure was near normal. Two weeks later with 33 pounds of stored fat gone forever, my blood pressure was perfectly normal; it has been since. It is obvious the condition of obesity was responsible for the blood pressure rise when combined with constant pain and sleeplessness. The stress of not being able to practice my chosen profession likely played a part in the scenario as well. Losing weight brought my blood pressure back to normal, despite the fact that nothing else had changed.

Why, when we are eating, do we consider eating so much food quickly? Why do we take such large mouthfuls of food? Why does the slow process of weight gain seem to be ignored by the gainer? Do we have to eat the whole bag or box of food? Do we have to drink volumes of calorie-containing liquids? Wholeheartedly answer these questions based on what you are learning in these pages.

I hope you understand when at an all-you-can eat buffet or a holiday meal, there is literally no limit to how much food you can eat—until your stomach tells you how miserable you feel from eating too much food. You have to be aware of your calorie intake, and you must do all you can to control your calorie intake at every meal and snack. You must be consistent. After a day of failure occurs, two days of strictness in this plan will put you right back on track.

Minimize the setbacks, and your accomplishment will be rapid. Remember an occasional day of failure is normal and expected. If this occurs once every two weeks or less often, you will be amazed at how your newly-found methods to lose unwanted pounds work for you. The weight scale does not lie. Your rapid progress will motivate you to continue, communicating with others will give you strength where you were once weak, and teaching a friend or relative will encourage you to finish the task.

Undoing your past is an exciting process. Realize few things come easily in life. Realize vigorous exercise will burn calories and tone muscles—all good—but will not compensate for too high a calorie intake. Realize it is the taste of food you enjoy, not the volume. Realize nutrition comes from sources other than food and drink. Realize commitment comes from within; not from someone else.

Realize healthy rapid weight loss takes you to your goal weight one time, and one time only. The mountain will never have to be climbed again. Once you learn how to accomplish the feat, weight maintenance is a small rollercoaster of molehills. You proved you could do it. Weight maintenance is a matter of respecting and trusting your knowledge. Learn well. Realize your philosophical, psychological, and physiological characteristics need to be in synchrony with each other to succeed. Realize the empowering qualities of making it to Z. Stay focused, and undo your past.

variation in wardrobe

Without question, a significant loss of weight will change your size and shape. As pounds are lost from losing body fat, you will notice your clothing getting looser on your body.

If you have clothes in storage at home that used to fit nicely, then you should utilize them as you continue to approach your ideal weight. I am a pack rat. I keep things from my past—items I may never use again. However, the clothing I stored came in handy as my body's size continued to shrink.

When I began the quest to lose 52 pounds, I wore size 40 waist pants. At that time my 40s were too tight. I didn't want to move up to the next size. My belt was on the last hole available. Thinking back on thinner days, I had a 32 inch waistline when I was a senior in high school.

In the beginning of week six, I dropped my calorie intake range again, 800 to 1000. Three days later, I dropped range from that level to 700 to 900 calories daily. By the end of week six, I had lost seven more pounds for a six week total of 40 pounds—only twelve pounds to go in two weeks to reach my goal of 180 pounds.

I refused to buy new clothes at that time, knowing I wasn't to my target weight yet. The last thing I wanted was to invest in new clothing that would be of inappropriate size in the near future. I didn't measure my waistline. I comfortably wore size 36s from my past clothing supply. It was simple math to calculate I had lost over 4 inches from my waistline so far, and I expected to lose additional inches as I finished the task. The holes in my belts which had not been used before were a welcome discovery. Things were very much in my favor mentally at this time. I was determined to finish what I had started—on time.

People around me consistently noticed changes they saw in my size. My students were making excellent progress as well, commenting in their emails how excited they were to be accountable to me and to themselves regarding the concepts of Z. Their bodies were changing in size as well. The committed students were experiencing the early stages of what I experienced. My results were reproducible in them. They were following my advice and understanding the nature of the truths I shared with them. We were getting smaller as we stayed strict with this plan.

ways to win

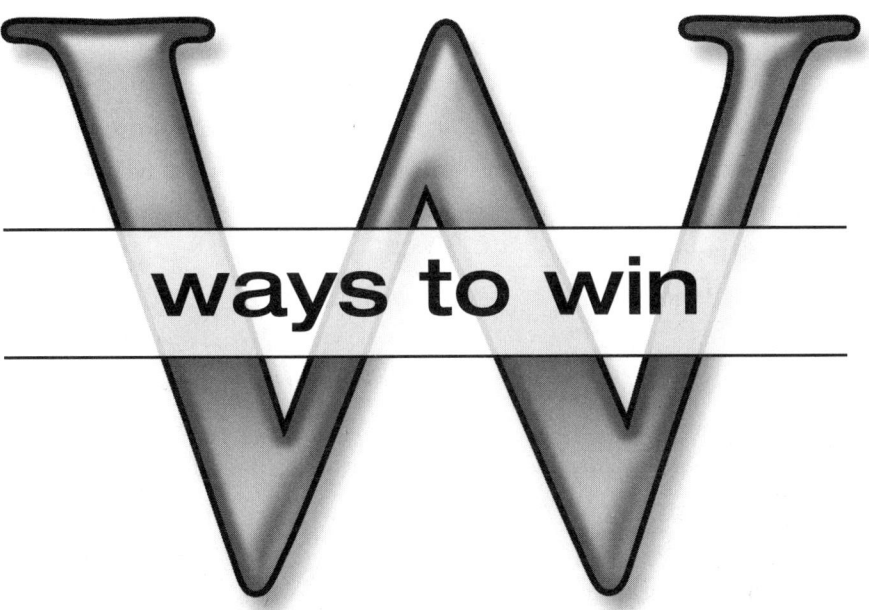

Everyone needs guidelines in their lives, whether for education, tax assistance, professional advice, tips on raising children, or weight loss.

In an attempt to take you to a healthy weight, I remind you it does not require a large investment of money. My approach is to minimize costs as you succeed in your quest. Do not continue to spend your money on false promises or on profit-driven programs that string out approaches, keeping your hard-earned dollars going in their direction. Save your money for more concrete purposes.

These comments are intended to help you overcome your weight problem, spending as little money as possible to reach your goal. I have not spent time or money investing in weight loss products, but I can imagine what others have

z the ultimate resolution starts now

spent looking for easy answers to what they perceive as impossibility. It doesn't have to be that way.

I will teach you to overcome your weight loss struggle, and I will include more than getting to your goal as part of what I consider winning strategy. You will be affected for life if you learn well.

I have vaguely presented information regarding daily calorie ranges, thus far. By saving the best for last, you will be encouraged in these last chapters to maximize the power of your own inner strength, and realize the benefits of a renewed, realistic perception of rapid healthy weight loss.

Calorie ranges in this program are as follows:

1300 to 1500 (starting range)

1200 to 1400

1100 to 1300

1000 to 1200

900 to 1100

800 to 1000

700 to 900

600 to 800

500 to 700

400 to 600

As you can see, there are ten calorie intake ranges present. Each represents a staging level of at least three to four days. Staying in a specific calorie range daily allows your stomach to adapt to a new level of "normal." This pattern continues each time you drop to the next calorie range. This being true, in about five weeks (on day 37), you could be in the lowest range if you drop range every four days. If you drop your range every three days, you will be in the lowest range in four weeks (on day 28). If you drop your range once every week, you will be in the lowest range after nine weeks. Drop your range once a month and you will be in the lowest calorie intake range in nine months. Which do you think would lead to rapid weight loss? Which do you think could provide the most motivating results in your case? Why will you take all recommended nutrients every morning after weighing in and recording the number?

I consider getting to your ideal weight quickly not only as being a healthy possibility, but also as being the most rewarding approach for you personally. What you will commit to for a relatively short period of time will transform you into a different person. I am not thinking about the obvious changes that will occur in your physical shape and size. Your perspective, your outlook on life, how you feel about yourself, and many other parts of your psychological makeup will undoubtedly be fine-tuned to your advantage.

For women of child-bearing capacity, starting weigh in is the third night when menstrual flow starts. Weigh yourself at bedtime. Go to bed hungry that night. Record your weight in Appendix A. All other committed candidates should pick a specific night to start; be sure to go to bed hungry that night after recording your bedtime weight. You

z the ultimate resolution starts now

cannot be hungry when you are sleeping.

When you step on the scale the next morning, record the number in your chart. Do this for at least four weeks, as outlined in Appendix A. Pay particular attention to the blurbs of text in that appendix. Each tidbit of advice is relevant. I would not have included these things otherwise. Some comments will cover familiar ground. The material is added intentionally to bring significant points to your attention as you record personal information each day. They are simply stepping stones to your success.

Your bedtime weight at each one week interval will be your weekly progress. If you wish, make a continuing document of your progress from start to finish. It helps you stay accountable, and teaches you what I recommend are true facts. The format I chose worked fine for my information, and for information I gathered from others I have taught. Record your early progress. You will kick start the motivational process as you see your accomplishment unfold quickly. You will likely want to continue recording your progress. I did, and I learned from it.

I must share the story of someone special, someone whose progress in this plan is notable to say the least. I will address her as "my friend." She wishes to remain anonymous at this time. This story has moved me to tears as it unfolded. I have told this one many times. I am so pleased I could help her.

My friend and I already knew each other professionally. At one of my follow up examinations on her turf, she saw me and wondered how I lost so much weight. I told her I designed the plan as a desperate measure to help my back problems, and I would be glad to show her how I was losing weight. Computer interactions started at once. She purchased the low-priced nutritional supplements I recommended. Wal-Mart has a wide variety and an affordable selection of vitamins, minerals, and antioxidants. She was on her way.

My friend lost 10 pounds in week 1, even with a day of failure on day 6. She was not in a premenstrual water retention phase, but she ate above her range that day. The next morning she weighed more than the morning before. This was merely a day of failure. She still lost 10 pounds in the first week. I was very pleased.

In week 2 my friend was motivated by that day of failure on day 6, and was determined to be strict. Her calorie range was dropped to 1200 to 1400 on day eleven, since she had been eating an average of 1300 calories per day up to that time and was making excellent progress.

The myth that the first ten pounds a dieter loses is all water weight loss is inaccurate. I, as did she, drank gallons of water during the first week, and all weeks to follow. Dehydration is unhealthy and well-respected in this plan. Drink as many zero calorie drinks as you desire. Drink small amounts of caloric liquids just for the taste. Drink at least eight 8-ounce glasses of calorie-free liquid every day.

My friend's calorie range was dropped again when she was comfortable at her previous range. On the morning of day 14, her range was adjusted to 1100 to 1300 calories per day. She had 1105 calories of intake that day. Comparing her bedtime weight on day 14 with her starting bedtime weight two weeks before, she lost 21.5 pounds in the first two weeks! No exercise regimen was recommended; she was advised to carry out normal daily activities, minus overeating. This remains the two-week Z record currently, taking my 18 pounds out by three and a half pounds. We each had one day of failure in the first two weeks—but only one. Remember that.

On the nineteenth night in week three, I advised lowering her range again to 1000 to 1200 calories per day, and she responded accordingly. The bedtime weigh in at three weeks set another record, that being 30 pounds. My dear friend lost another eight and a half pounds in week 3; an unbelievable, but true story.

I recommended she stay in that calorie range until further notice, and she did well. The week 4 record she holds is 36.5 pounds lost. The week 5 record she holds is 42 pounds lost.

On the second day of week 6 her range was dropped—900 to 1100 calories per day. At the end of week six, she still held the record at 41.5 pounds lost. She ate less that week, but gained one half pound. Premenstrual symptoms started the day before her 5 week record was set. She was not progressing while eating less. I predicted it would happen. It will happen with all women of childbearing capacity. Week seven was stable—no gain or loss. This is perfectly normal under these physiological circumstances.

On the morning of week 8, I recommended a drop in calorie range again; down to 800 to 1000. Into three days of flowing monthly visitor activity, my friend's scale numbers dropped like a rock as before. Adult female water retention phenomena ceased. Rapid healthy weight loss resumed. From her Tuesday night to Sunday night weigh in numbers, she lost nine pounds in five days for a week 8 total of forty nine and one half pounds. She was well on her way to her goal at that time. This friend had lost 49.5 pounds, comparing her eight week bedtime weight with her starting weight—just eight weeks earlier.

When my friend saw her mother and some other close family members for the first time in two years, she was eager to share her secret with them. She had lost 73 pounds at the time. She had lost over 23% of her total body weight. Her family members did not know she was losing weight.

Her doctors recommended my friend have her stomach stapled less than a year earlier, but her insurance wouldn't cover it. She was told morbid obesity would lead to her death in 7 to 10 years if she did not lose weight. She tried everything in the past with no success.

I present information derived from email communications we have had as I mentor her:

"I have been having problems with my scale. It seems to be inconsistent."

She recorded her initial weight at bedtime on her starting date, and she went to bed hungry. She was in the recommended starting calorie range—1300 to 1500 calories. The next morning, she weighed 1.5 pounds less than the night before. My friend strived to stay in her calorie range on day one. On the 2nd morning, she had lost an additional two pounds.

"Is that normal? My calorie intake yesterday was 1289 (not quite 1300), I took my multivitamins and drank all my water. I did not eat after 7:30 and I went to sleep with my stomach growling."

My response included, "I think your scale is totally correct. It is your friend. Will not lie to you."

More from my friend:

z the ultimate resolution starts now

"Do you want to hear something that has given me even more motivation?"

At her bedtime weigh in on the 3rd night, my friend had lost 6 pounds. The next morning, she was down another pound. She had lost seven pounds by the 4th morning.

"Put it this way, the sun is shining and it isn't even up yet."

"I feel as if I had a great day."
On her 12th night, she had lost 16.5 pounds.
"I am happy to say I had my highest calorie intake at breakfast and worked my way down from there. Dinner was at 7:30 this evening. My calorie intake was 1340 today, 900 of which was before 4:00 p.m. I feel so positive today and even have more energy."

On her 19th night, my friend had lost 26 pounds.
"Great Day...I am soooooo motivated. Good Friday has been a good Friday for me. I feel as if I have the world on a string, and I am in total control. I have not felt this good in years. You are my mentor, my friend, and my guide to a world I have not been a part of in over 25 years. In the back of my mind I can see that person and I like the way she looks. Today's calorie intake was 1174. I am so excited, and I owe it all to you. Thank you."

"Six months ago I would have never thought this was possible. In fact six months ago I was scheduling myself for gastric by-pass surgery. Can you believe that? I was grasping at my last straw because I felt it was my only hope to see my 50th birthday. The only reason I did not go through with it was that my insurance would not pay for it—for weight loss surgery due to obesity."

"I thought the 800-1000 range would be tougher to stay in between. So far, it has been a lot easier than I thought. More people are noticing my weight loss. Just subtle comments are being cast my way, like "You've lost a chin," or "I can see your waist," or even the old standby, "Have you done something different to your hair?" I love it because they are so used to me eating they haven't realized the obvious—that I am not. Oh, before I forget, yesterday's calorie intake was 824."

"I never thought I would ever eat under 1000 calories and still be able to function. You are right; it is amazing. If someone would have told me I would be eating like this a few months ago, I would have told them it was impossible. I still cannot wait to see what my mom thinks when she sees me. She has no idea I have been doing this."

At exactly 73 pounds lost, my friend visited her family.

"I have to tell you that when I stepped off the plane (my mom met me at the airport) mom did not recognize me at first. She actually took a double take. She couldn't believe how good I looked; we both cried. Bill, you cannot imagine the emotions that continued to flow out of me every time I saw another relative. They were all amazed and excited for me. I even have three nieces and a couple of friends that want me to mentor them when I am able to."

"When one of my brothers saw me he actually ran up to

Z the ultimate resolution starts now

me and picked me up, hugged me tight, and told me how proud he was of me; yes, again I cried. He told me he had to pick me up because when he hugged me, he was able to get his arms completely around me for the first time in years. As I said, he was so proud of me. This trip was the best thing that has happened to me in a long, long time."

I thank my friend for believing in herself, believing in mentorship, and believing in change.

This program changes lives, not lifestyles. Please continue to customize your perspective. Search for and learn ways to win. Follow all recommendations contained in Z; not one of them is to be omitted from your sound advice list if you plan to succeed. Plan to succeed, and be totally committed on your very first attempt.

x-treme results are possible

If you are intentionally shrinking your stomach regularly, then there is no need for surgical intervention. There is no need to risk post-surgical complications. Absolutely no hardware is necessary. Using the basic physiological concept of adaptation, we train our stomachs to adapt to a specific amount of food intake. In three or four days that very thing takes place. Our stomachs adapt to the new level of food intake quickly, and less food intake over time continues to be enough. In my opinion, a rumble in my tummy during the race was a good sign. It was a sign that I was winning; that I was on my way to accomplishing something special. The word special cannot begin to describe what reaching a challenging goal can do for a person.

As one enters the lower calorie ranges of this program,

one continues to adjust the thought processes. Protein intake of twenty grams a day is recommended. This is not an all-protein, all-low-carb, or all-low-calorie foods plan. However, I do recommend sufficient protein intake daily for optimum health during rapid weight loss. Good protein sources are not hard to find: meats, fish, nuts, peanut butter, etc. I personally chose deli-shaved ham, almonds, peanut butter, beef, chicken, and seafood as high-protein elements of my diet. What I ate is not the relevant point: you will eat only what satisfies you. Look up the numbers. Consistently be aware of what focused attention on these numbers represents: optimum health during rapid weight loss.

Remember these during your journey: daily nutritional supplements, accurate account of calories consumed each day, adequate water intake, and daily protein gram intake. Each is of major importance. Calorie content of each serving must always be respected to maintain accuracy of your daily intake. Stay in your calorie range every day as you plan meals and snacks. Eating twenty grams of protein every day is a must for your health as you progress to your goal. Your daily vitamin, mineral, and antioxidant supplements are absolutely necessary. They provide a wealth of your nutritional daily needs; however, they do not supply necessary daily protein. Pay strict attention to these facts. Remember starvation does not play a role in this plan; your supplements, water intake, and protein intake prevent it from being possible if you have excess body fat to burn.

Play an intelligent role in this process; extreme results come from extraordinary efforts.

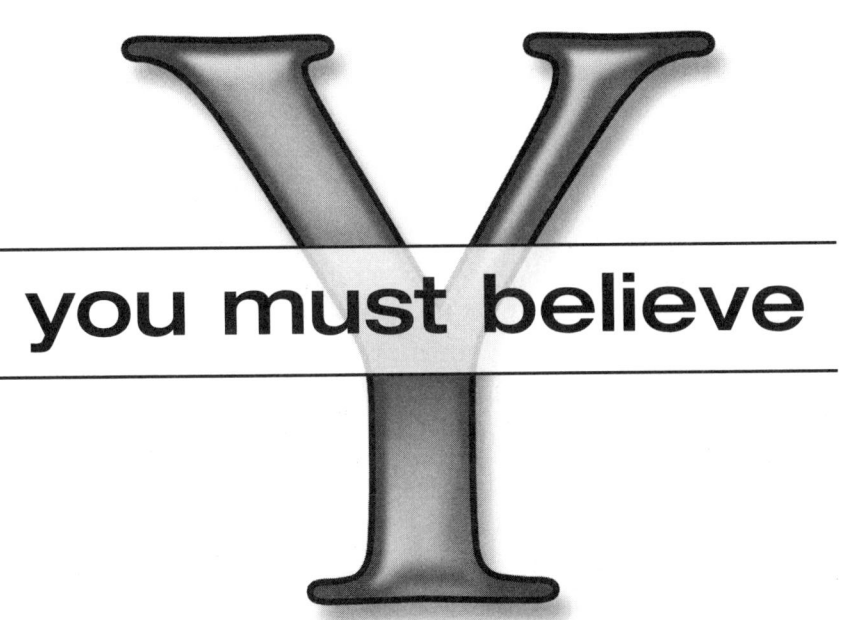

you must believe

If you can't do it, nobody can. I you can do it, everybody can. I believe anyone who is truly committed to losing weight can. I believe encouragement is powerful. I believe that loneliness leads to failure. You must believe strength comes in numbers. Communication with others is extremely important to your success. Let people know you are committed to reaching your ideal weight. They want you to win.

You may be on the computer during communication with others. If you know your mentor personally, this is a good thing. If you don't, keep your identity anonymous. Don't fall in love with your mentor. I do not want people sharing good information with each other to be infiltrated by sickos or pranksters out there. Always be careful when communicating by computer. Unfortunately, there are scammers and

Z the ultimate resolution starts now

sociopaths in our world. Be aware of this, please. Identify them, report them, and avoid them. Try to communicate with people you already know, or a truly qualified Z mentor.

As defined previously, a mentor of this program must be at least 50% to his or her goal of reaching an ideal weight. I will identify with these mentors, and I will be the only person qualified to dub one a Z mentor. Finishing a quest as you inspire others keeps your motivation at its highest possible level. Email me personally at hbhop.com for mentor guidance or to report a problem, if necessary. I could end up being your mentor. I enjoy teaching people what I have learned and I will do everything I can to see to it that everyone has an opportunity to engage in these concepts.

I want to mentor in all 50 states with this plan, and watch it spread like wildfire—to other countries. I have mentioned obesity is a global problem, haven't I? I have to ponder the possibilities. My friends keep asking me in jest, "When are you going to be on Oprah?" I would be willing to go on if invited, without hesitation.

As I rapidly approached my goal, I dropped calorie range again in the beginning of week 7— 600 to 800 calories. Again, 3 days later, I went down another level to 500 to 700 calories maximum daily. My stomach wasn't complaining any more than I was accustomed to. I continued to eat three meals a day and snacked; eating lesser amounts of my favorite foods and drinking plenty of 0-calorie fluids before and after all meals. I did not ingest any calories after suppertime, and went to bed hungry every night. I lost six more pounds in week 7, and had a firm grip on planning week 8. The people I mentored continued to progress well, and I continued to refine a universal approach to rapid healthy weight loss as I charted our successes and failures.

Early on in communications with my sister Terry, she relayed thoughts to me concerning non-insulin dependent diabetes mellitus (Type 2 diabetes). I quote her from saved email:

> "I take 2000 mg of Glucophage a day. It wreaks havoc on my digestive system..diarrhea most every day. I know several other people that have the same problem from this med. It is my DREAM to be med free and control my diabetes through diet. I know it's possible...and it's a goal I'm striving for. My fastings have never been under the 90's since being an adult. Anyway...I'm just looking forward to great overall health...I want to feel great and get the bonus of looking great too!"

Visit the American Diabetes Association web site sometime. You will find the following information, I quote from their site, in the *All About Diabetes* section, subheading *Major Types of Diabetes:*

Type 2 diabetes
Results from insulin resistance (a condition in which the body fails to properly use insulin), combined with relative insulin deficiency. Most Americans who are diagnosed with diabetes have type 2 diabetes.

Pre-diabetes
Pre-diabetes is a condition that occurs when a person's blood glucose levels are higher than normal

but not high enough for a diagnosis of type 2 diabetes. There are 41 million Americans who have pre-diabetes, in addition to the 20.8 million with diabetes.

In the same location mentioned above, Type 1 diabetes accounts for 5-10% of Americans who are diagnosed with diabetes. Let us do the math. At 10%, of the 20.8 million quoted above, only 2.08 million of these afflicted are Type 1 diabetics (body fails to produce insulin, requiring daily injections). The other form of diabetes mentioned, gestational diabetes, accounts for about 135,000 cases in our country annually. About 4% of pregnant women develop this usually temporary condition.

Just a little more math. Based on the above numbers, about 18 million Americans suffer from Type 2 diabetes. Another 41 million people in this country are diabetics waiting to happen, pre-diabetics. These together total close to 60 million people of the United States. Roughly 70% of us are overweight or obese. Do you see a correlation there?

My question is how many pre-diabetic individuals would have normal blood glucose levels if they were at their ideal weight? Here is another inquiry I just have to mention. How many Type 2 diabetics would have normal blood glucose levels if they were at their ideal weight? My guess would be in the millions. I personally know two, so far. Derek is one of them. He is the first person to combat Type 2 diabetes by realizing and committing to the concepts of Z; reaching his ideal weight. Period. Not "just lose about 20 pounds, or so."

I was Derek's Z mentor. He followed my advice well. He went the distance without a copy of this book. He restored his health, and he lost a total of 62 pounds in his quest to better health, meeting his goal weight face to face in very good time.

Week 8 of my experience took me to the 400 to 600 calorie range. I ate 600 calories for two days, 500 calories for two days, and 400 calories for three days. The last range in this program finished the task. I stayed in range and got the job done. I ate three 100 calorie meals and two 50 calorie snacks for the last three days only. I would never have believed it was possible to reduce calorie intake so drastically and maintain ideal nutrition if I hadn't experienced it myself. Amazing? I do think so. Compare these numbers to the numbers in chapter D, page 13, second paragraph from the bottom:

ATKINS 2000	**Z 2005**
33 pounds in 14 weeks	52 pounds in eight weeks
	(33 pounds in five weeks)
avg: 2.36 lbs/week	6.50 lbs/week
avg: 1.01 lbs. every 3 days	2.79 lbs. every 3 days

In all examples above, doing the math again, Z was nearly triple the efficiency of the diet plan I utilized in the year 2000. When I finished dieting in that year, I was still 20 pounds overweight, and happy to weigh "only" 200 pounds.

I did lose the last six pounds in week 8. I weighed 180 pounds on Sunday night, March 13, 2005 at bedtime. Eight Sunday nights before I was 52 pounds heavier. The lofty goal I set for myself was met, with hope that maintaining a healthy weight would ultimately have a positive effect on my failing back.

z the ultimate resolution starts now

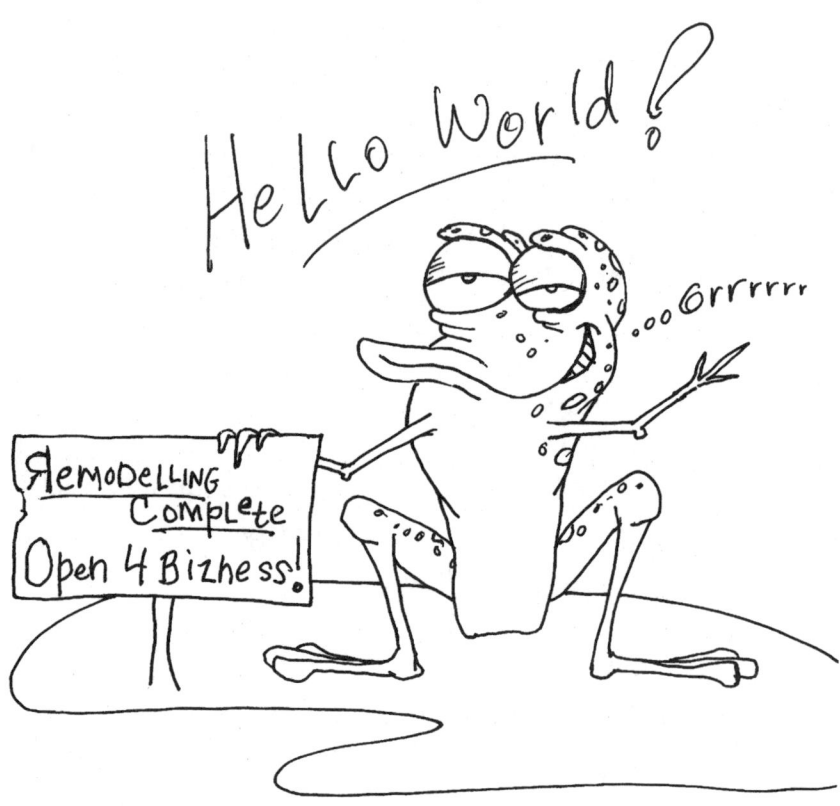

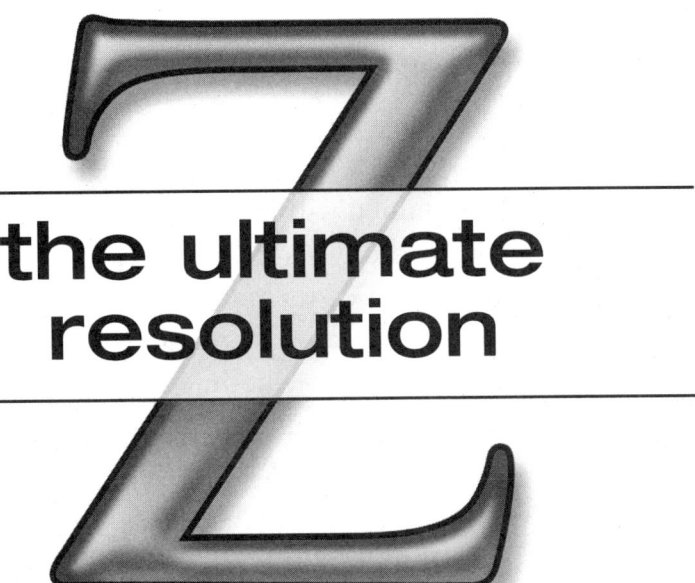

the ultimate resolution

A resolution requires determination. If you are determined to succeed and you learn well, then you will succeed.

Most people trying to lose weight are not motivated as I was—by an attempt to regain physical normalcy for my career's sake and my family's sake. It is interesting I would have never tried to lose weight quickly otherwise. This plan was discovered from pure circumstance. What I did resulted in progress like nothing I have ever heard of; it was, and is, my intention to spread this advice as far from Bowling Green, Kentucky as I can. The first stage of this commitment is in my home country, the United States of America. I will reach out with this book to as many people as possible. When good news spreads by word of mouth, it is far-reaching. As I have mentioned before, global coverage is part of

Z the ultimate resolution starts now

what I perceive as possible.

Z is a plan and a place. It is the ultimate resolution.

It does not have to be January 1st when you commit to this program.

The plan is contained within this book's covers. No plan can be carried out without performance. Use the information and the recommended techniques contained between this book's covers to your advantage. Do not forget what you learn. It will be important for lifetime weight maintenance.

Communication by computer can enhance your potential for success. If you cannot, or do not use a computer, commit to all information in these pages. Try to access a computer at your local library if you can, and learn to communicate by computer. Share what you are doing with other people. Do not be alone. Solitude in a struggle can lead to deeper struggle.

The mysterious place called Z is where you will be physically, emotionally, psychologically, and philosophically when you reach your ideal weight. It is truly mysterious; the changes that will take place in you are unknown currently. These changes are unique to you as an individual.

You are a success waiting to happen. Be totally committed to reaching your ideal weight before you start. Be committed to reaching that weight as quickly as you possibly can.

Z is rapid healthy weight loss. Maintaining or improving your health during this process is not unlikely, it is the norm. I contend the overall health of Z participants reaching their goal is likely to improve. It is not a possibility. It is a probability. People who are overweight or obese will probably be in better overall health if they reach their ideal weight. One could boldly replace the word probably in the last sentence

the ultimate resolution   z

with the word definitely. People who are overweight or obese will definitely be in better overall health if they reach their ideal weight. This comment is the most realistic.

I believe it is important for anyone who is trying to lose weight to understand eating disorders. The National Eating Disorders Association has an official web site. Please look up what they have to say to gain additional perspective. The keyword *neda* is used if you have computer access. Access the NEDA web site and scroll down to find *Eating Disorders Info*. Using some of this information can help you understand the intricacies of these significant mental health problems.

I must add here that all information in the NEDA web site cannot be recommended in this book. Obese and overweight individuals should not be encouraged to stay in their unhealthy physical condition, or let anyone lead them to believe their condition is healthy.

The following quotes come from NEDA in the above italicized section of their web site:

kNOw Dieting:
Risks and Reasons to Stop

"Americans spend more than **$40 billion dollars** a year on dieting and diet-related products."

"Dieting has become a **national** pastime, especially for women..."

"Dieting rarely works."

"Dieting forces your body into starvation mode."

"Dieters often miss out on important nutrients."

"Dieting can lead to an **eating disorder**."

"Next time the dieting desire crosses your mind, take a time out. Think about the reasons why you want to lose weight. Are they really worth it? Think about the potential dangers of dieting."

In your best interest, compare every statement above with what I recommend in this book. Ask yourself the following question: What are the potential dangers of not dieting? Getting to your ideal weight is not only on of the healthiest things you can do for yourself, but also it is one of the most life-transforming things you can do for yourself. **Is it really worth it?** The answer is definitely yes. Why any group would recommend overweight or obese individuals maintain an unhealthy weight is beyond me. That certainly is not what the medical profession recommends as ideal for overall health, and it certainly is not what the American Diabetes Association recommends for overall health. I can guarantee that.

Exercise is good for the health of your body, your mind, and your heart. I mentioned earlier I could not exercise vigorously during the time I lost weight. I could float around in a swimming pool and move my legs. I could swim slowly. I could walk carefully, but not without pain. I was physically restricted from nearly all forms of exercise. This does not mean I do not recommend exercise. I do, and I wish I could exercise vigorously. It *does* mean vigorous exercise is not required to reach your ideal weight. If you can, I recommend light walking and swimming as the best exercise strategy for the overweight and obese population. Exercise alone will not result in weight loss if overeating is part of your daily routine.

You may be wondering what one does to maintain his or her weight once an ideal weight is reached. Let me explain to you exactly what I did once I reached my target weight of 180 pounds.

Since I was only eating 400 calories a day for three days when I reached my goal, I realized the prediction that I would have to increase my calorie intake. I knew my stomach had adapted to a very small size as I meant it to, so I gradually increased my daily calorie intake. Every three days I increased my calorie intake to the maximum of each intake range on the chart. I started with 600 calories for three days, then 700 calories for three days, et cetera, reversing the process that led to success. Thirty days later I was eating 1500 calories a day. I was intentionally stretching my stomach to the size I reduced it to during the starting days of this plan. My stomach was too full for a month, and I realized how senseless it was to overeat so routinely in my past. My weight stayed stable during that month, fluctuating within a few pounds of my goal weight as I increased my caloric intake. These actions prevent additional weight loss once one has reached his or her goal weight.

Depending on your metabolic rate and amount of exercise in which you engage, a stable weight can be maintained with a consistent calorie intake around 2000 calories. Your goal for the rest of your life is to never be more than 10 pounds over your ideal weight in the future. Do not go back to overeating daily. If you do over do it on a particular day,

z the ultimate resolution starts now

you should already know two days of less than normal calorie intake will offset the gain. Use what you learned during healthy rapid weight loss to your advantage. What was a mountain to climb initially is now a series of barely significant molehills. Fluctuate within ten pounds of your ideal weight for the rest of your life. There will be no health risks relating to obesity. You are always close to or at your ideal weight if you do what I recommend above. If you get out of control and gain 20 pounds, reinstitute Z. You should not have to do this if you learned well and discovered self-control during the process of getting to your ideal weight the first time. You should only need to find Z one time. From that point forward, pay strict attention to the good habits you have learned, and minimize your past bad habits. Eat and drink sensibly. Keep your stomach a consistent size for the rest of your days. Live in the reality of Z.

Epilogue

As one makes the commitment to reach his or her ideal weight, one must institute changes in eating behavior regardless of external or social pressures. When you focus on an effort to lose weight quickly, try to block out or avoid interferences in your pathways to success. It does not matter how others around you are eating. You can eat however you intend to eat when you are in public.

If you go to a restaurant, for example, keep your eating habits under control. I had no problem eating less than I used to at a restaurant. You must learn to avoid the one thousand calorie basket of rolls or breads placed in front of you. Have some bread if you like, but pay strict attention to your serving size. Move the basket to the other side of the table if necessary. Drink zero calorie drinks. Order whatever you like, including dessert. If you like salad, ask for your dressing on the side. Lettuce is a low calorie food. Dip your fork in the salad dressing, and then pick up the lettuce. This is much better for your calorie control than allowing your salad dressing to drench your entire salad. Do the little things that make a difference. Every bit of effort helps. Ask for a take-home container before your meal comes. When the meal is served, do your magic. Take your meat portion and divide it into thirds. Put two thirds of it in the box. Do the same with all high-calorie foods on your plate. Make sure you leave some of each item on your plate; control the portion size specifically for all foods in the meal. Put what you are not planning to eat in the take-home container. Take your time enjoying the taste of the foods you choose. Don't be embarrassed to use small bites in front of others. Do what produces the best results and still satisfies your taste buds. It is your way of enjoying the meal maximally while eating less. Focus on the dining experience, not the availability of food. Enjoy your company and the surroundings. Leftover food from the restaurant will continue to feed you in the coming days. You save money on groceries while getting the most for your money when dining out. You get three meals for the price of one.

Can you control yourself at an all-you-can-eat buffet? Most people cannot. We try so hard to get our money's worth. Overeating is the result. I avoided buffets for eight weeks. I did not purchase the opportunity to overeat during that time. I knew it would be a barrier to rapid weight loss. I did go on a weekend men's retreat in week three. There were buffet breakfast, lunch, and dinner opportunities that weekend—four of them to be exact. There were also plenty of snack foods, including candy bars, in the hall where we gathered.

I ate candy all day long, but tiny amounts at a time—just for the taste. I ate at the buffet breakfasts, lunch, and dinner as well. I served myself small portions of many foods, ate like a mouse in the presence of other men, and lost 2 pounds while I was there. Remember my motivation to lose weight in a specified amount of time. It can be done. During the eight week period in which I lost fifty two pounds, I drank about 200 calories of liquid. I insisted on not wasting potential food calories on drinks. It was to my advantage.

Eat consistently each day. Three meals a day is the optimum pattern, with snacks between meals. Minimizing or eliminating calorie intake after suppertime will allow you to

epilogue

go to bed hungry. I cannot stress the importance of this. Going to bed hungry will motivate you to have breakfast the next morning. A consistent intake of food and drink each day satisfies your stomach. I was happy to go to bed hungry. I slept through hunger, and woke up with predictable weight loss. Staying in specific calorie ranges along the way allowed my stomach to adapt optimally to less food intake over time. You do not have to eat less and less forever—just until you quickly reach your goal weight. Once my ideal weight was reached, I quadrupled my daily calorie intake over a period of five weeks to gradually readapt my stomach to larger amounts of food intake over time. I reversed the program so I would not continue to lose weight. This approach made perfect sense to me and produced optimum results. I still overdo it sometimes. I respond by eating less than normal for two days. It evens the score, and a healthy weight is maintained long term. I let my size 34 waist pants motivate me to pay attention now. If my 34s are a little tight instead of a little loose, I take it easy on calorie intake for a few days. I lost a total of seven inches from my waistline on my way to Z.

Now it is your turn, my friend. You have the information you need to reach your ideal weight in a relatively short period of time. It has been my pleasure to share with you. I hope you enjoyed the read as much as I did the write. Now that you have read these words from beginning to end, I hope you are ready to take on the challenge of getting to your ideal weight. I hope you do it in good company and in minimal time. I hope you are truly committed to this plan, honest with yourself, knowledgeable of the techniques, strong in spirit and determination,

z the ultimate resolution starts now

and confident that you can do almost anything if you put your mind to it. I feel certain your inner strength can overcome your past weakness.

Are you ready? Are you committed to being strict and going to a place you have never dreamed of going quickly? Are you confident this program has promise like no other weight loss program you have ever seen? I sure hope so.

Z, the ultimate resolution, starts **now**. Be persistent and be prepared to succeed.

Appendix

_____'s Weight Loss Chronology

Weekday/Date	Weight/Calories	(Go to bed hungry every night)
_____	B _____ (start)	**B** = bedtime (before sleep)
_____	M _____	**M** = morning (before taking supplements with 0 cal. drink)
_____	B _____	
_____	M _____	*Women with regular menstrual cycle: initial weigh in is 3rd night of menstrual flow at bedtime.
_____	B _____	
_____	M _____	Starting weight is at bedtime on your chosen start date. Be committed.
_____	B _____	Record M and B weights each day; Record daily calorie intake after B weight every day after start date.
_____	M _____	
_____	B _____	Weekly progress is calculated by subtracting bedtime weight of the same weekday as starting night (each week) from the starting night weight.
_____	M _____	
_____	B _____	*(Sun. 1/16 B weight minus Sun. 1/23 B weight, for example)*
_____	M _____	
_____	B _____	You may use blank spaces in chapter text for note taking or jotting down calories consumed for each date. Add daily totals and record after B weight on that date. Keep track accurately.
_____	M _____	
_____	B _____	

Week One Progress: _____ pounds

Note: Above includes starting night weigh in number and seven full days of space to record Week One: M and B weights, with room for total calorie intake each day to be recorded next to B weights on that date. This allows you to monitor progress from day to day, and from week to week. Note your calorie range in margin. Start in 1300 to 1500 calorie range initially. Drop calorie range down one level every three to four days for optimum results. "Staple" your stomach a little at a time.

Special note to women of child-bearing capacity: Commonly in week 3, you will notice a halt in rapid progress. This is normal and is expected. Stay in your pertinent calorie range as recommended, or drop range if you are doing well at your current range. That is, you can drop range every 3 or 4 days if you wish. Do not expect that change to make a big difference in weight loss progress until your 3rd day of menstrual flow. Rapid weight loss will resume at or near that time.

acknowledgments

Thank you to all early participants I mentored in this program. Through information recorded in my database via our interaction, I had a wealth of pertinent material at my fingertips. These facts were analyzed as correspondence continued, allowing the concepts contained herein to be fine-tuned for the advantage of others who seek to lose weight with this healthy rapid approach. Your feedback provided so much more information for me to go on than just my own journey to Z. It proved reproducibility in others, as well. May what we have learned be used to help many others overcome their pain.

With deep emotion, I would like to thank the following men and their families for financially supporting the birth of HBHOP Publishing Company: Mark Kiernan, Dr. Eric Ladd, Dr. Jeff Jordan, and Dr. Carl Newton. I have known each of these men as friends for at least twenty years. In a very difficult personal struggle with total disability, I was lifted up by their generosity and support. HBHOP would not exist without the help of these true friends.

I would like to thank Dave Owens, a college apartment mate at Indiana University, Bloomington. His doodling and unique cartooning ability has been entertaining me since 1982 when we met for the first time. Our friendship continues to last. This man's talent goes far beyond what you have seen in these pages. Dave Owens, better known as the Random Variable to me, is truly a one-of-a-kind artist. I realized his ability many years ago, and predicted he would be famous one day. It is my wish to see much more of his work come to full fruition in the near future.

Thanks to Bill Kersey of KerseyGraphics in Nashville, TN. Your patience and kindness has made this career-changing experience a blessing. Your talents are treasure. Meeting you and working with you was like communicating with a long-time friend.

Thanks to everyone at Vaughan Printing Company in Nashville, TN. I appreciate your efforts to help me thrive in such unfamiliar territory. A special thank you goes to Jean Leasure for her one-on-one communication with me, her advice, and her expertise. You made what could have been difficult much easier to manage.

Finally, thanks to you, the reader. With perseverance and commitment to this program, I hope you find what you long for. I hope this book is the final piece you need to solve a difficult puzzle. Please do your very best to learn what I teach and teach what you learn. It is my prayer that you reach a healthy weight as quickly as you can, and that your efforts are rewarded with a longer, healthier life.

All these words come straight from my heart.

Dr. Bill Hopkins